Orthopaedic Surgery for Students and General Practitioners: Preliminary Considerations and Diseases of the Spine; 114 Original Illustrations - Primary Source Edition

Robert Tunstall Taylor

DEDICATED

TO

EDWARD H. BRADFORD, M.D.

AND

WILLIAM OSLER, M.D.

EARLY FRIENDS AND ADVISERS

PREFACE.

In the following pages, the author has endeavored to provide a text-book for his own undergraduate students, which would be of sufficient brevity not to strike terror to the "fourth-year-man," who is taxed now with numerous specialties, and at the same time to make it sufficiently exhaustive to permit of application and to cover the most modern and accepted views of the subject. No attempt has been made to write an extensive treatise on orthopædic surgery, nor have statistics, numberless references and obsolete methods of treating individual deformities been cited, but methods only, as a rule, which have proven useful to the author.

Baltimore, March, 1907.

CHAPTER I.

Orthopædic surgery is that branch of the surgical science
which has to treat of the nature, cause, prevention, or
correction of deformities by gymnastic, mechanical or surgical means, or all three. In early times, hernia, strabismus
and tumors of various kinds, were by some included within
the scope of orthopædic surgery, but the term is now given
chiefly to the consideration of diseases or deformities, which
involve the bones or the articulations. Formerly the term
was restricted to the correction of deformities in children
from the derivation (ὀρθὸς, straight and παῖς, child), but is
now extended to all ages. It is more frequently misspelt
"orthopedics," which the derivation does not warrant and
leads many even in the profession to the belief that it treats
of deformities of the feet chiefly, mixing the Latin "pes,"
"pedis," with the Greek word "παῖς," "παιδίς."

As a special branch of surgery, orthopædics may employ
in treatment hygiene and physical culture, using out-of-door
life (tent dwelling), gymnastics, Swedish movements, massage and electricity; surgical operations, which allies it with
general surgery, but does not invade, but amplifies that
domain; medication to supply deficiencies in the economy
of the organism or combat pathological processes; dietetics
to insure proper feeding and to correct vicious conditions,
such as malnutrition, rickets and scurvy, due to errors in
the quantity, quality, temperature, preparation and character of food; and mechanical appliances and apparatus to aid
functional use, to overcome faulty attitudes and malposi-

tions, to preserve proper alignment, to exercise traction or fixation on the extremities and spine.

Orthopædic surgery as a specialty separated from general surgery is of comparatively recent date in America, for its first chair dates from 1861, when the elder Sayre filled it at Bellevue Medical College. Now forty-five of our American medical schools announce special instruction in this branch, showing the widespread recognition of its importance and but few state board examinations omit questions on this subject.

From the earliest times, however, descriptions and methods of treatment of deformity have been found in surgical literature.

Nicholas Andry of Lyons, who lived from 1658 to 1742, and became a surgeon in Paris, wrote on orthopædic surgery and originated the name "L'Orthopédie." Many have called him the "Father of Orthopædic Surgery," but treatises on this subject are of much earlier origin, for they have been found as far back as the writings of Hippocrates, the "Father of Medicine," who lived 460–370 B. C. and his monographs show that he had some very good methods in treating deformities, considering the period in which he lived. In his article "Concerning the Articulations," he wrote of the treatment of "club-foot,"[1] to be spoken of later. He also wrote of spinal affections and "tubercle within and without the lungs." In the "Hippocratic Writings"[2] of the Greek schools of Cos and Cnidos, which probably embrace not only the work of Hippocrates himself and his pupils, but also the methods and views of his predecessors, are found accounts of the articulations, of

[1] The genuine works of Hippocrates translated from the Greek, by Francis Adams, M.D., London, 1849. Published by the Sydenham Society, vol. ii, pp. 632–662.

[2] J. S. Billings: History and Literature of Surgery; Dennis, System of Surgery, vol. i, ch. 1.

traumatic and congenital dislocations, especially of the knee, elbow and ankle joints, methods of reduction and of apparatus.

Some specimens of Jewish surgery are to be found in the Talmud, where it is shown that they knew of the application to the body of artificial parts, viz: wooden legs and apparatus of various forms for unfortunates, who were deprived of the use of their lower extremities.

In the literature of India are found two medical works, the "Charaka" and "Susruta," the date of which compositions is variously estimated at from 1000 B. C. to 700 A.D. In the translation of "Susruta" by Anna Moreshvar Kunte, published in Bombay in 1877, we find in subdivision five, the "Koumarabhrityam," which treats of the care and treatment of children and the use of appliances for them.

The first treatise on surgery was written in Rome by Aulus Cornelius Celsus, "the Medical Cicero," who lived about the beginning of the Christian era. He was more of an author of an encyclopedia or compiler of the arts and sciences for literary men, than a physician, and introduced many Greek words for which he could not find a Latin equivalent. He speaks of dislocations of the head of the femur and many kinds of machines for extending the femur after reduction.

Claudius Galen, who was born at Pergamus, 131 A.D. and finally settled in Rome, is said to have written some five hundred treatises on medicine. His "De usu partium" contained much anatomy and in his writings are also found a description of the section of the sterno-cleido-mastoid to correct torticollis and a method for the radical cure of hare-lip.

Ætius Amidenus of Constantinople, a Christian, who lived in the early part of the sixth century used word-charms and for removing sequestra in osteomyelitis recommends the following: "Bone, as Jesus Christ caused Lazarus to come out of the grave, as Jonah came out of the whale's belly, come out," a method which we of today find quite unavailing

Paul of Ægina, the last of the Greek medical writers, who studied at Alexandria, lived in the early part of the seventh century and most of the Arabian physicians received their inspirations from him.   He wrote seven valuable books on medicine.   In fractures of the spine and spinous processes he says, "having first given warning of the danger, we must, if possible, attempt to extract by an incision the compressing bone."

Albucasis of the Arabian school, who died about 1105 A.D., wrote in his third book of fractures, luxations, sprains, etc.

Gui de Chauliac born about 1300 A.D., settled at Avignon, wrote in his "Great Surgery," as it was called, "up to the time of Avicenna all writers were both physicians and surgeons (i. e., well educated men), but since that time, either because of fastidiousness or the excessive occupation of the clerics, surgery has become a separate branch and has fallen into the hands of the mechanics."   It is to be supposed this was a slur, just as later the orthopædic surgeons by ultra-conservatism, were called "buckle and strap men," by their critics.

Ambroise Paré (1517–1590), who increased the standing of the corporation of barber surgeons although a great military surgeon and devoting so much of his time to gun-shot wounds, devised several orthopædic methods and appliances, notably the brass cuirass for spinal disease.

Paracelsus (1493–1541) contributed some little to the treatment of deformities, but his writings were chiefly given over to the care of wounds.   It was he who wrote that "some surgeons use the probe merely because they have seen it used and to show that they are doing something."

Hendric Von Roonhuysen (1625–1626?), of Amsterdam, operated for hare-lip and wry-neck.

The "Leech Book," written about 970 A.D., is the oldest English medical book and in it we find, "For hare-lip pound mastic very small, add the white of an egg and mingle as thou dost vermillion; cut with a knife the false edges of the lip, sew fast with silk, then smear without and within with the salve, ere the silk rot. If it draw together, arrange it with the hand; anoint again soon."

Another remarkable account of an operation in England in the seventeenth century is found in the "Diary of the Rev. John Ward, vicar of Stratford-upon-Avon" (1648–1679), in which he says: "The mountebank that cutt wry-necks cutt three tendons in one child's neck, and hee did itt thus; first by making a small orifice with his launcet, and lifting upp the tendon, for fear of the jugular veins, then by putting in his incision knife and cutting them upwards; they give a great snapp when cutt. The orifice of his wounds are small, and scarce any blood follows."

Francis Arcæus (1493–157?), a Spanish surgeon, described an apparatus for the treatment of club-foot and advised mercurial inunctions on the joints for syphilis, which disease had been first described by John de Vigo, an Italian surgeon, in 1514.

We now come again to Nicholas Andry (1658–1742), dean of the medical faculty of Paris in 1724, who is known in medical literature chiefly by his book, "L'Orthopédie, où l'art de prevenir et de corriger dans les enfans les difformités du corps" (Paris, 1741), being the first work in which the term orthopædic is used.

Jean Louis Petit (1674–1750), of the same period, first described mollities ossium.

"The practice of medicine was forbidden to the executioners in Prussia, but in the year 1774 Frederick the Great granted to them permission to treat fractures, wounds, and ulcers and when the Berlin surgeons complained of this, he issued an order saying that he had not permitted all executioners, but only the skillful ones to practise and if the surgeons are as skillful, as they pretend to be, everyone will rather trust them than go to an executioner; but if the surgeons are ignoramuses, the public must not suffer, but must submit to be treated by the executioner rather than to remain lame and crippled."[1]   According to this, today the orthopædic surgeon has taken the place of the executioner.

The foremost English Surgeon at this time was Sir Percival Pott (1713–1788).   He became surgeon to St. Bartholomew's Hospital in 1749 and published in 1779 his "Remarks on that kind of palsy of the lower limbs which is frequently found to accompany curvature of the spine."   This was the first accurate description of the gross lesions of humpback, which disease still bears Pott's name.

John Abernethy (1764–1831), Pott's successor at St. Bartholomew's, introduced an improved method of opening lumbar abscesses "to admit the least possible amount of air."

Henry Park (1774–1831) of Liverpool, a pupil of Pott and Le Cat, has his name linked with resection of the knee and elbow, and Charles White of Manchester first excised the head of the humerus in 1768.

Among the English surgeons who wrote of joint and bone diseases may be named Sir Benjamin Collins Brodie (1783–1862), who wrote "Pathological and Surgical Observations on Diseases of the Joints," in 1818; William Ferguson (1808–1877), who devised the term "conservative surgery" in sparing all of limbs possible in bone disease by excisions; James Syme (1799–1870); Edward Stanley (1791–1847); George M. Jones (180?–1861) excised the hip, knee,

---

[1] J. S. Billings: Dennis, System of Surgery, vol. i, ch. 1.

ankle and scapula; Joseph Sampson Gamgee (1828–1886) devised starched apparatus for fractures and joint disease; Abraham Colles (1773–1843), whose name we use in speaking of fracture of the proximal end of the radius and "Colles' law" of syphilis. W. J. Little, himself club-footed and a patient of Stromeyer's (v. i.), published valuable treatises on club-foot (1837–1839), and "Deformities of the Human Frame" in 1843.

Robert Adams (1791–1861) wrote of chronic rheumatic arthritis; Robert William Smith (1807–1873) of congenital dislocations; Henry Hancock (1809–1880) of the foot and ankle joint; John Cooper Forster (1823–1886) of the surgical diseases of children; Peter Charles Price (1832–1864) on excision vs. amputation in knee-joint disease.

In France we find writings by Guillaume Dupuytren (1778–1835), after whom the contraction of the tendons and palmar fascia is named, and who wrote of congenital hip dislocation and subcutaneous tenotomy of the sterno–cleido-mastoid; Philip Joseph Roux (1780–1854) on cleft palate; Jacques Lisfranc (1790–1847) on partial amputation of the foot; Jacques Mathieu Delpech (1777–1832), who pointed out that Pott's Disease of the spine was of tuberculous origin, and in 1816 first performed tenotomy of the tendo achillis for talipes equinus, following a Dr. Lorenz's operation at Thilenius' suggestion on a patient of the latter, which was later popularized and applied to this and other tendons by Georg Friedrich Louis Stromeyer (1804–1876) of Hanover in 1831.

Moritz Gerhard Thilenius (1745–1809), of Frankfort on Main, was the first on record, who proposed division of the tendo achillis for talipes.[4] Others of his time and even subsequently blamed the distorted tarsal bones and not the tendons for the primary deformity. On a patient of his,

---

[4] Adams: Club-Foot. Lindsay & Blakiston, 1873.

a girl of fourteen, on March 26, 1784, a surgeon by the
name of Lorenz divided the tendon "on which the heel
immediately descended two inches, enabling the patient to
tread on the entire sole. The foot was retained in its
improved position by appropriate bandages and the cicatrization of the large wound was complete on the twelfth of May.
The cure was so perfect that the patient walked as well as a
sound person." Following this case Sartorius operated on
a case of equinus in a boy of thirteen who had had abscesses
on the "back of the leg" six years previously (probably from
a tuberculous ankle). He dissected out the tendon through
an incision four inches long, then divided it. Great force
was necessary to correct the deformity (from evident ankylosis at the ankle), and Sartorius was much censured for this
forcible correction, although "the result in nine weeks was
satisfactory."

Michaelis in November, 1809, operated on his first case
"by dividing the tendon one-third through and immediately
corrected the deformity." He subsequently operated on
seven other cases. As previously stated Delpech in May,
1816, made a punctured wound (the first attempt at subcutaneous tenotomy) of an inch on either side of the tendo
achillis in a boy of nine years, divided the tendon from
within out with a second knife, corrected the deformity and
then manually tried to bring the severed ends of the tendon
together, applying fixative dressings, as his idea was that
union would be more satisfactory if the deformity were later
corrected mechanically while the lymph was "still soft and
possessed ductility." As it happened the case suppurated
and "indolent abscesses were formed on the inside of the
leg, the inside of the patella and in the inguinal region; and
neither these nor the wounds from the operation were healed
for some months." The patient was ultimately cured, but
Delpech did not record another case of tenotomy but laid

down the rule that "the tendon should not be exposed, but section should be done by a circuitous route."

Fifteen years later Stromeyer, in February, 1831, made a much smaller puncture with a tenotome on a case, endeavvored not to puncture the skin on both sides, although he said it did not matter. He did not believe in immediate but subsequent correction of the deformity by mechanical means, a foot stretcher and Scarpa (Antonius Scarpa, 1747–1832) shoe, and on this case and 150 more he succeeded and made the operation permanent.

Others of the same period who wrote of joint surgery were, Alfred Armand Louis Marie Velpeau (1795–1867), whose bandage we use in clavicular and shoulder joint conditions; Amédée Bonnet (1802–1858), who made useful studies in spinal and joint diseases; Charles Gabriel Pravaz (1791–1853), who first put orthopædic surgery on a scientific basis; Jean Gaspard Blaise Goyrand (1803–1866), who wrote of loose bodies in the joints; Jules Roux (1807–1877), who first made use of iodine injection into the shoulder joint; Henri Ferdinand Dolbeau (1830–1877), who contributed to our knowledge of club-foot and spina bifida, and Joseph François Malgaigne (1806–1865) of dislocation and fractured patella.

Jules Réné Guérin (1801–1886), the founder of the Gazette médicale de Paris specialized in orthopædic surgery and established a private sanitarium. His first book on deformities appeared in 1838 and in 1882 the "Oeuvres du docteur Jules Guérin," etc., which were to fill sixteen volumes were started, but never finished. He was more popular as a critic and writer with the laity than the profession.

In Germany we find Johann Friedrich Dieffenbach (1792–1847) practicing orthopædic surgery in 1832; Michael Jaeger (1795–1838), who wrote largely of diseases of bones and joints;

Friedrich August von Ammon (1799–1861) devoted much attention to deformities; Bernard Rudolph Konrad von Langenbech (1810–1887), who broadened surgical knowledge in nearly every department; Carl Hueter (1838–1882), who wrote treatises on joint diseases in 1870 and 1876; Theodor Billroth (1829–1894) threw much light on surgical pathology, and Richard von Volkmann (1830–1880), one of the founders of the German Surgical Association, devised the bone curettes known as "Volkmann spoons."

In this country much was added to our knowledge of orthopædic surgery by Dr. Nathan Smith of Yale (1762–1829), who first used a trephine in osteomyelitis and introduced manipulative means to reduce dislocation of the hip joint; by Dr. Wm. C. Daniel of Savannah who first employed extension by weight in the treatment of fracture of the femur; by Dr. J. Kearny Rodgers (1793–1851) of New York, who did an osteotomy in ankylosis of the hip in 1840, following Dr. John Rhea Barton (1794–1871) of the University of Pennsylvania, who first performed this operation in 1826.

Thomas Dent Mutter (1811–1859) of Virginia, later of the Jefferson Medical College, added to our knowledge of plastic operations to correct deformities following burns.

Henry Jacob Bigelow (1816–1890) of Harvard excised the first hip joint in this country in 1852.

Gurdon Buck (1807–1877) of New York popularized the treatment of fractures of the thigh by weight and pulley, which is now so much used in contractures, especially in muscle spasm in tuberculous disease of the spine, hip and knee joints, and known as "Buck's extension."

Alden March (1795–1869) of Albany made valuable investigations of hip disease.

John M. Cornochen (1817–1887) of Savannah wrote on congenital dislocations of the head of the femur. Robert Alexander Kinloch (1826–1891) of Charleston, S. C., who was medical director on the staffs of Generals Lee, Pemberton and Beauregard in the Civil War, first successfully in this country excised the knee for chronic disease.

Henry C. Davis devised the traction splint for tuberculous hip disease and the antero-posterior support for Pott's Disease.

Along with the introduction of anæsthesia in 1846 by Drs. John Collins Warren (1778–1856) and Henry Jacob Bigelow (1816–1890) of the Harvard Medical School (after Dr. Crawford W. Long of Athens, Ga., in 1842, and Dr. Morton, a Boston dentist, had independently produced insensibility by ether), and the introduction of antiseptic and aseptic surgery by Sir Joseph Lister in 1867, on the basis of Pasteur's experiments, which proved that putrefaction is due to the action of microörganisms, orthopædic surgery partook of the general new life infused into surgical practice and became more and more specialized and operative in the nineteenth century. Bigelow published a "Manual of Orthopædic Surgery" in 1844, and he may be regarded as the father of this specialty in America.

More recently the names of Buckminster Brown of Boston, James Knight, Louis A. Sayre, who made the plaster bandage and jacket popular and Charles Fayette Taylor of New York stand out as laying the foundation upon which has been built the American School of Orthopædic Surgery and the results of whose teachings are found in the Transactions of the American Orthopædic Association, which was established in 1887. These Transactions today represent the most original, advanced, suggestive and thorough work done in this specialty in America and are now published as the American Journal of Orthopædic Surgery.

The late Dr. William Detmold held private clinics at Bellevue Hospital, New York, in this specialty as early as 1841, and in the New York Medical Gazette, January 1, 1851, vol. ii, we find an editorial to the effect that, "Dr. Detmold has consented to deliver a course of lectures on orthopædic surgery, a department in which he has long been distinguished and the importance of which can scarcely be overrated." However, regular orthopædic work was not begun at Bellevue Hospital, until Louis Albert Sayre was appointed visiting surgeon in 1853. In 1861, Bellevue Hospital Medical College was organized and the first chair of orthopædic surgery was established with Dr. Sayre as professor, as has been noted in the beginning of this historical sketch.

The first special institution for the crippled was advocated by Dr. James Knight in New York as early as 1842, but it was not until 1863, that the valuable Hospital for the Ruptured and Crippled of New York City was finally incorporated with Dr. Knight as surgeon-in-chief, although for twenty years he had specialized in orthopædic surgery and was noted for his philanthropy.

Dr. Charles Fayette Taylor, the then consulting orthopædic surgeon to St. Luke's, established the New York Orthopædic Hospital in 1866. The Boston Children's Hospital, which is one of the most thorough and advanced institutions for the treatment of deformity existing today, was incorporated in 1869, chiefly through the efforts of Drs. Francis H. Brown and William Ingalls.

CHAPTER II.

SURGICAL SUPPLIES, INSTRUMENTS AND NECESSARY APPARATUS.

As orthopædic surgery requires a special equipment not usually found in a general surgical armamentarium, it may be well to go somewhat into detail in regard to certain appliances and supplies which should be at hand to facilitate work.

THE PLASTER OF PARIS BANDAGE.

Perhaps no one thing, if properly made of suitable materials, is more useful and constantly needed in orthopædic practice than the plaster bandage and nothing more unsatisfactory than one which does not set properly, is gritty, heavy, lumpy or thick.

A wet plaster bandage should feel, before application, smooth, uniform and of the consistency of very soft putty.

Naturally the elements that enter into a good bandage are the crinoline, plaster of paris and the mode of preparation and keeping. The ordinary crinoline found in ladies' furnishing stores is not suitable for making plaster bandages as it contains glue, which will not mix properly with plaster and retards setting; but the crinoline should be made with starch only.

Sometimes one finds in hospitals plaster of paris bandages made of cheese cloth or ordinary surgical gauze or of dressmaker's crinoline with the glue washed out, but none of these are as satisfactory as the starch crinoline named.

The plaster of paris which will be found the best is that known as dental plaster, to be had in any of the larger cities from druggists and to be purchased in tins, kegs, half-barrels or barrels. Of course, the last measure, when much is to be used, is the most economical, provided the barrel is emptied into tin cans or buckets with air-tight covers to prevent moisture from causing the plaster to become air slaked before use. · This is a most important essential to success with bandages and even when bought in 50 or 100 pound tins, one need not expect to obtain good bandages if the tin is left open for moisture to get at the plaster or if a damp rainy day is chosen as the time for making bandages. After the bandages are made they should be kept in air-tight tins until used. It is an unnecessary refinement to wrap each plaster bandage in oiled paper, for those, over a year old, loose in a covered tin, have been found perfectly satisfactory.

The crinoline comes in pieces, of course, and can be torn in strips, three inches (9 cm.) wide and about four to five yards (3–4 m.) long for general use, being made somewhat narrower for bandaging small children's feet and wider for plaster jackets and spicas in adults. These strips are rolled loosely.

To prepare a bandage about 18 inches to 2 feet (60 cm.) of one end of the strip of crinoline is drawn out on a table, previously covered with a piece of mackintosh, on which half a pound or so of the plaster of paris is poured. Then with an ordinary table knife or spatula a uniform, thin layer of the powdered plaster is spread on the crinoline to a thickness of .5 to 1 mm. With the left hand, the finished portion is loosely rolled up and a new area drawn out, while with the right hand holding the spatula an additional area is spread with the powder. As each bandage is finished it is to be placed in a covered tin, until used.

Various machines have been devised for making plaster of paris bandages, but none have proved to give the quick-setting, uniform bandages made by the method described. Many machines present the fault of allowing moisture to get at the plaster.

When bandages are to be used, various suggestions have been made, such as adding salt to the water or using hot water to promote quick setting, but these are unnecessary and uncomfortable to the patient and tepid water answers every purpose, insuring a bandage setting not too quickly and not too friable when set as is the case when salt is added.

Authorities differ as to the best method of placing the bandage in the pan of water, which should be of sufficient depth to well cover the bandage, but the author has found laying them flat and not on end, insures a more even distribution and speedy saturation, which can be determined, when the bubbles cease to rise. But one or two bandages should be put in the water at a time, otherwise some will set before use.

To wring the bandage grasp with a hand over each end to keep the plaster in and squeeze out the surplus of water. Some surgeons preferring rather a dry bandage and others one that is rather moist.

As each turn of bandage is carried around a part, it should be well rubbed, and smoothed out with the hand to insure an even distribution of the plaster in the meshes of the crinoline and promote setting.

The plaster being spread on one side only of the crinoline, a plaster of paris bandage cannot be reversed, as can the gauze or muslin bandage, but in order to accomplish the same result, it can be reduplicated on itself or cut through and started in a new direction.

When a cast is completed it can be rendered more smooth by moistening the hands several times and rubbing in the plaster more thoroughly, or a muslin bandage can be moistened and drawn backward and forward across the surface until polished and smooth. Perhaps the best finish to the surface can be given, just before the plaster is finally set, by rubbing with a round smooth bottle and a little water.

In applying plaster, ordinarily it should not be applied directly in contact with the skin, since the hair becomes caught in the plaster and thus causes discomfort on removal and since the hard plaster erodes the skin over bony prominences.

A seamless stockinet is made and sold by the yard and in sizes to permit of application to the extremities or trunk as a foundation for plaster bandages, but when this is not at hand a very snug-fitting undershirt or thin stocking may be used.

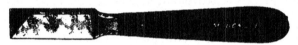

FIG. 1. PLASTER KNIFE.

At times when allowance has to be made for swelling of the soft parts, cotton batting, to be had at drygoods stores in sheets, with a glaze on both surfaces, is to be used after tearing it into bandages three or four inches (9 cm.) wide and rolling it for convenience of application.

Not infrequently it is essential to comfort, that the bony prominences under a plaster dressing should be unusually well padded to prevent sloughing of the skin and for this purpose piano-felt is the best material to use. Pieces of this felt can be cut off in suitable shapes as needed and sewed on the stockinet to protect the points desired.

The vast majority of plaster dressings put on by the ignorant or unskilled are found to be three or more centimeters in thickness, often cruelly heavy for small children. A properly made and applied cast should not be thicker uniformly than from three to eight millimeters or at most one centimeter for the heaviest adult patient, unless it is to be worn for a very long time.

Much has been written and said about the supposed difficult task of cutting off a plaster cast, some suggesting the softening of the plaster by means of hydrochloric acid, vinegar, etc., when in reality it is a very simple process not requiring any of the complicated and numerous instruments devised for the purpose. But three things are needed, a

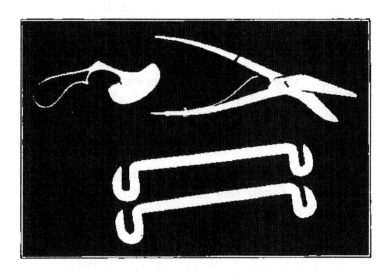

FIG. 2. PLASTER SAW, SHEARS AND BRACE BENDING IRONS.

sharp, short-bladed, square-end knife like a glazier's, a crescent shaped thin saw and a medicine dropper. (Figs. 1 and 2.)

To open a plaster dressing make a straight shallow cut with the knife down the proposed opening and with the medicine dropper fill this cut or scratch with water from time to time, and it will be found that a straight clean opening can be made readily with the saw, down to the stockinet or cotton batting. When one has cut through the plaster to the foundation it is easily determined by the difference in sound with no danger of scratching the patient. The stockinet is then best cut by ordinary bandage scissors.

At times a pair of plaster shears will be found useful to trim plaster jackets and spicas in the axillæ and groins.[6]

TRACTION STRAPS AND APPLIANCES.

To apply Buck's extension to the legs for fractures, dislocations, hip disease, tuberculous knee disease, contractures following paralysis, burns and rheumatism, acute Pott's Disease and Pott's paralysis, we have two methods best adapted to accomplish it, viz: the two and five-tailed method of strapping. The materials used consist of webbing from one-half to three-quarter inch (1-2 cm.) wide, ordinary surgeon's plaster and what is known as swansdown adhesive plaster, as less irritating to the skin and stronger than the ordinary plaster.

To make the two-tailed traction strap, two strips of adhesive plaster are taken one inch (3 cm.) wide and of the approximate length of the patient's leg, *i. e.*, from the anterior superior spine of the ilium to the internal malleolus. To one end of one of these strips about six inches (18 cm.) of webbing is sewed and the second strip of adhesive plaster is sewed at this junction at an acute angle of 45° to the first strip. A similar strap is made for the other side of the leg with the angle reversed. (Fig. 3.)

To apply the two-tailed traction straps, place the junction of the adhesive strips and webbing about two inches (5 cm.) above the malleoli with the oblique piece of adhesive forward and the straight pieces as near the middle of the sides

[6] The plaster knife, saw and shears, as well as other instruments, braces and bed attachments mentioned in these notes, can be had of J. D. McGonigle & Co., 1125 East Baltimore Street, Baltimore, Md.

of the leg as possible, where they are to be stuck. In sticking it to the thigh it is well to pull the skin down a little before sticking it to gain as much as possible when the traction is made. Then the oblique straps are wound spirally around the leg and thigh without tension. To com-

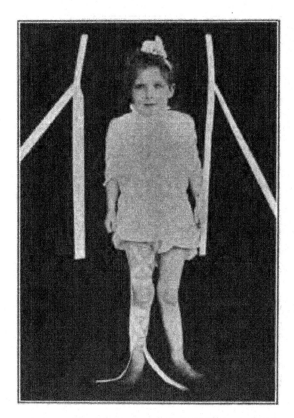

FIG. 3. BUCK'S EXTENSION TWO-TAILED STRAPS.

plete the bandage turns of adhesive three-fourths of an inch (2 cm.) wide are put around the ankle, calf, lower and upper thigh. To insure thorough adhesion between the skin and plaster the whole is covered by a gauze bandage, preferably with one ragged edge turned in for neatness, put on spirally.

To make the five-tailed traction straps, which are to be preferred, the swansdown adhesive is to be used as it is stronger and less irritating. A strip six inches wide and of the length of the leg is cut. This is cut into two pieces for the two sides of the leg, as follows; two inches (5 cm.) is

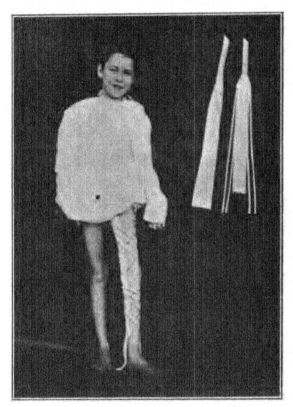

Fig. 4. Buck's Extension Five-Tailed Straps.

measured on one end and a division is made to a point two inches (5 cm.) from the diagonally opposite corner, so that each piece will be two inches (5 cm.) wide on one end and four inches (10 cm.) wide on the other. (Fig. 4.)

A tail one-half inch (1.5 cm.) wide is now cut down each side to within two or three inches (10 cm.) of the narrow end.

Then two tails are cut to extend an inch from the knee and two or three inches (10 cm.) of the remaining middle portion is cut off to reinforce the narrow lower end, to which the webbing is now sewn. The central tails are stuck to the middle of the side of the leg with the lower ends two inches above the malleoli; the four lateral tails remaining on each side are wound spirally upward, as in the two-tail method and the whole covered by a bandage.

All adhesive plasters should be kept in a cool place. The paper on the swansdown adhesive if stuck tightly can be removed with a sponge moistened in water.

To remove adhesive straps from the skin they should be well moistened with alcohol or benzine and will then be found much more easily taken off without pain. In adults the leg should be shaved before adhesive straps are applied.

THE SPREADER.

What is known as a "spreader," to keep the webbing straps from pressing on the malleoli, is a curved piece of steel, having a loop in the center and a buckle screwed to each end. In these buckles the webbing is fastened and in the loop a stout cord, preferably the white plaited kind, is fastened. The other end of the cord passes over a pulley at the foot of the bed and on its other extremity the weight is attached to exert traction on the leg. A spreader can be made of wood with buckles, bits of leather and a picture loop. Buck's extension traps should be changed every two weeks to prevent excoriation of the skin.*

THE INCLINED PLANE.

An inclined plane is sometimes needed, while traction is being made, to support the leg (almost invariably in hip disease) where the ilio-psoas muscles by their spasmodic con-

* R. T. Taylor: Trans., American Orthopædic Association, vol. xii, 1899, p. 355.

traction produce a flexion of the thigh on the body. The inclined plane should be so made, that it can be raised to any desired angle up to 60°, for by this adjustability traction can be made "in the line of the deformity" and be adapted to the degree of contraction of the ilio-psoas muscles or to

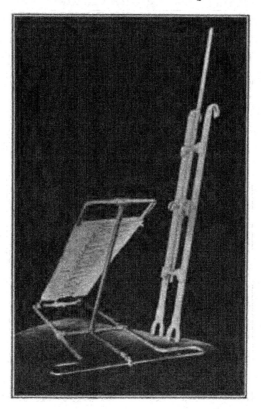

FIG. 5. AUTHOR'S TRACTION ROD, PULLEY AND INCLINED PLANE.

such a position that would tend to facilitate the traction on the tense muscles when in their most relaxed condition.[7]

THE TRACTION ROD.

In order to make traction in the line of the deformity, which is most essential in several conditions, it is necessary

[7] *Ibid.*

to have the pulley at the foot of the bed adjustable to best accomplish the desired aim and the author has devised a steel traction rod with adjustable pulley and also the steel inclined plane frame which can be covered with a twill cotton cover to be laced on.

These are sterilizable in case the child has some infectious disease while being treated for some surgical trouble, which is not possible with the older wooden appliances, which of course can be made in emergencies.[a]   (Fig. 5.)

BED FRAMES.

This brings us to that most useful appliance, the "bed frame," devised by Dr. E. H. Bradford, of Boston, which is so very important in maintaining fixation of patients, when they are being treated for tuberculous disease of the spine, knee and hip, as well as fractures and other conditions requiring immobilziation of the patient.   It is quite ridiculous to go into some hospitals and see children being treated (?) for hip disease, sitting up in bed with the spreader in contact with the pulley and the weight on the floor, thus having the disadvantages of confinement in bed with none of the benefits hoped for.   (Fig. 6.)

With the Bradford bed frame the patient can be fixed on his back and in the case of the hip, traction can be made constantly in any desired direction.

These rectangular frames are made of gas pipe, varying in size with the patient, and are oblong and quadrilateral, being joined at the corners by "elbows."   When complete they are covered by two twill cotton covers which lace by means of eyelets on the under surface and can be changed when soiled.   Crossed straps of webbing which pass over the shoulder and under the axilla on each side and then around

[a] *Ibid.*

---

the frame, like military cross straps immobilize the patient. The pelvis is fixed also by a webbing strap, which passes over it and around the frame.

The frames to be satisfactory should fit the patient and can readily be made by any plumber. They should be

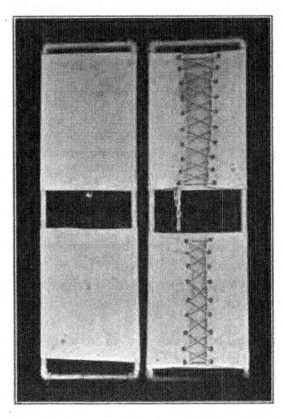

FIG. 6. BRADFORD BED FRAME.

four inches (10 cm.) longer than the patient and two inches (5 cm.) broader than the patient's shoulders. These two dimensions will give the desired size for the frame. Then to make the frame covers, measure from the top of the patient's head to the tuberosities of the ischium for the length of the upper frame cover and have it 1¾ times as wide as the frame. Allow an interval of four inches (10 cm.), then measure to bottom of the frame for the lower cover and make it also 1¾ times as wide as the frame. Along the edges, which are to go underneath the frame, there should be a double row of stitching and strong eyelets put in by a tent or sail-maker.

The interval of four inches between the upper and lower frame covers is left, so that a bed pan can be slipped under the frame, when needed, without disturbing the patient's

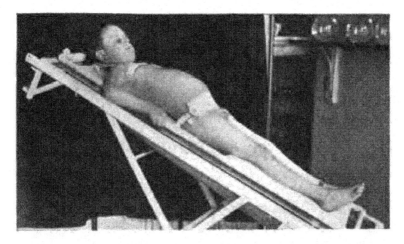

FIG. 7. AUTHOR'S METHOD OF FIXATION ON BRADFORD FRAME.*

position. These covers should be laced as tightly as possible in order that they may be very smooth, comfortable and *firm* to lie upon.

The author has devised an apron with buckles, clips and straps which are more secure in fixing patients on these frames than the cross straps ordinarily employed. The clips are sprung on the frame by a forceps and obviate the necessity for buttonholes in the frame covers. These bed frames possess the additional advantage of portability, are

* *Ibid.*

like small stretchers, so that ill patients can be carried out-of-doors into the sunshine and fresh air, the ends being rested upon chairs making thereby an improvised lounge, or carried to the operating room for dressings, etc., wherever immobilization is a desideratum. (Figs. 7, 8 and 9.)

Other frames have been devised, that of Phelp's being of wood board, cut the shape of the child's head, trunk and limbs. When padded the child lies on this board and is encased in plaster of paris, subsequently the front of the

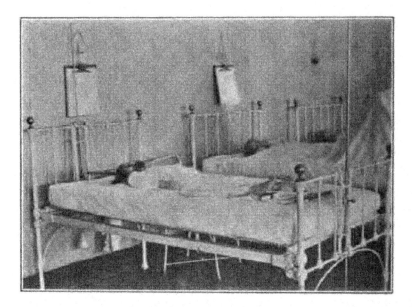

FIG. 8. THE BED TREATMENT OF VERY ACUTE POTT'S DISEASE WITH HEAD TRACTION, DOUBLE BUCK'S EXTENSION ON LEGS AND FIXATION ON THE BRADFORD FRAME.

plaster is cut away, so that the child is held in a trough. This is not as cleanly as the Bradford frame.

The Sayre cuirass, made of wire the shape of the patient's head, trunk and lower extremities offers the same objection and in addition is more expensive.

The instruments needed beyond the usual surgical equipment are but few, and consist of osteotomes, an osteoclast, a bone-hammer and tenotomes, And for brace work bending irons, vise, screwdriver, pair of pliers and leather punch. For records are needed a tape measure and piece of lead-tape. A camera and skin pencil are also useful for the same purpose.

The osteotomes which have been found most useful by the author are known as the MacEwen osteotomes. There are two forms of bone cutting instruments of the chisel order to be distinguished; one the osteotome, having both planes

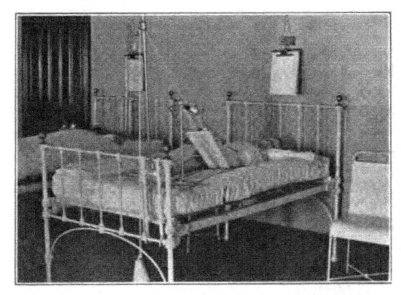

Fig. 9. Inclined Plane Used in Acute Coxalgia to Accomplish "Traction in the Line of the Deformity." Fixation is Obtained by the Bradford Frame.

gradually sloping down to a sharp cutting edge, the other made like a carpenter's chisel with one plane beveled off near the cutting end more than the other. The osteotome is like a long slender wedge and should have a temper between that of a cold chisel and a carpenter's cutting tool, so that the edge will not be turned by the hardness of the bone, but at the same time cut into it and not so sharp as the carpenter's tool or ordinary bone chisel for fear, in doing subcutaneous osteotomies, if the instrument should slip, there should be danger of cutting large arteries or nerve trunks. (Fig. 10.)

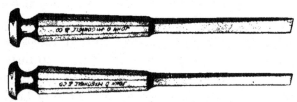

FIG. 10. MacEwen Osteotomes.

One should have two widths of osteotome one a half an inch wide (1.5 cm.) and one a quarter of an inch (1 cm.) in width for smaller bones. Each should be graduated in centimeters so that one could tell to what depth the instrument is driven in. It is most important that the planes should gradually approach the cutting edge and not have a sudden bulge just above the cutting edge for such an osteotome is apt to splinter bone. A large handle is also of advantage, as it can be grasped more easily and firmly.

The ordinary bone-hammer, as sold in the instrument stores, is unsatisfactory and noisy, being made of steel or with a lead head.

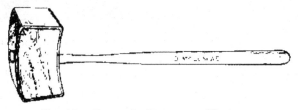

FIG. 11. Author's Osteotomy Hammer.

The best will be found to be the ordinary wood mallet, such as used for cracking ice or preferably a steel handle in a *circularly curved* wood pulp or lignum vitæ head, as was made for the author. (Fig. 11.)

OSTEOCLASTS.

For correcting bowlegs, a useful instrument is the Rizzoli osteoclast, by means of which a linear fracture can be made at any desired point without splintering. It consists of a steel bar through the center of which a triple screw passes with handle on one end and a padded movable steel plate on the other. This plate should be fastened to the screw by means of a swivel joint to permit of the adaptability of the padded surface to the skin. On either end of the main bar are padded rings, of sufficient size to permit the passage of

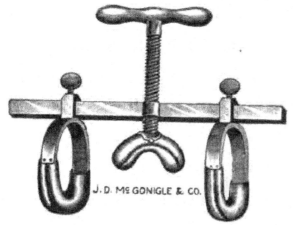

FIG. 12. RIZZOLI'S OSTEOCLAST.

an adult's foot and leg through them, with set screws to the bar, so as to be useful in all sizes and ages. (Fig. 12.)

The Lorenz osteoclast immobilizes the limb above the desired point of fracture in a kind of vice and by means of a strap below and screw the limb is fractured at the end of the vice. (Fig. 13.)

The Gratten osteoclast has a heavier screw than Rizzoli's, has a base of support and is much more powerful. (Fig. 14.)

The author's osteoclast depends on the lever principle, is more rapid and more convenient to use than the screw machines. It can be used to bend a softened and rachitic bone, as well as break a hard eburnated one. (Fig 15.)

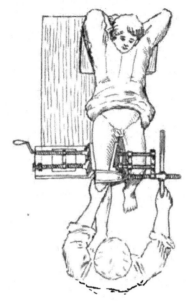

FIG. 13. LORENZ'S OSTEOCLAST. (Hoffa.)

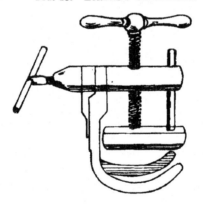

FIG. 14. GRATTAN'S OSTEOCLAST.

The instrument consists of a T-shaped base, surmounted by an arc holding an L-shaped lever and forward thrusting rod, which can be adjusted. On the end of this rod is a pres-

sure plate padded. Resistance is obtained by adjustable
C-pieces attached to the cross arms of the T. The adjustments
are aimed to accommodate differences in length, flexibility of
the bones and circumference in limbs.[10]

TENOTOMES.

Two or three tenotomes will be found all that are necessary, two being sharp on the point and one edge and having

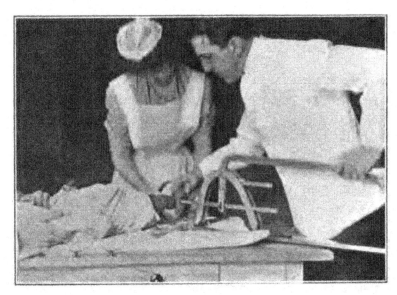

FIG. 15. AUTHOR'S OSTEOCLAST.

blades respectively one-half (1.5 cm.) and one-quarter inch
(1 cm.) long. The third should be blunt pointed with a
cutting edge on one side. (Fig. 16.)

BENDING IRONS.

Of the instruments needed for adjusting and fitting braces
the bending irons alone need description. They are steel

[9] R. T. Taylor: Amer. Jour. Orthopædic Surg., vol. xvi, p. 24, 1903.

rods one-half inch (1.5 cm.) square with rectangular hooks on
each end of different widths to slip over the steel uprights in
braces of varying sizes and by means of the handles enable
one to bend the brace as one would do with a pair of monkey
wrenches.   The edges of the hooks should be rounded to
avoid cutting the leather on the braces.   (Fig. 2.)

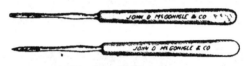

FIG. 16. TENOTOMES.

LEAD TAPE.

The lead tape, preferably an alloy of tin and lead, is about
one-sixteenth inch (2 mm.) thick, one-half inch (1.5 cm.)
wide and twenty-four inches (50 cm.) long, and is to be
used to mold over a part to obtain a tracing of it, using
the bent lead tape as a ruler.

HEAD SLINGS.

Head slings are devices to make traction on the neck or
spine and are made of webbing padded, of canvas or
leather, to go under the chin and occiput, usually buckling
just below the mastoid processes.   From the occipital and
chin pieces a strap passes to a ring above the head on each
side and to these rings a spreader is attached.   If the traction pulls the chin up unduly, causing extension of the head
additional straps can be fastened to the occipital piece for
attachment to the spreader.

CHAPTER III.

In no branch of medicine does skiagraphy play such an important and imperatively necessary rôle, as in surgery, where for diagnosis, in conjunction with the clinical symptoms, it is an invaluable aid. This is especially true in orthopædic surgery, where the bones and joints are the chief objects of investigation, which we have to examine thoroughly clinically in making our diagnosis.

On this account, it has been deemed wise to devote a brief chapter to X-ray apparatus and its mode of application, with no attempt to go deeply into the subject with electrical technicality and phraseology.

More comprehensive accounts of the subject are left to the special works on X-ray apparatus and technique and the reader is referred to such books as William's Röntgen Rays in Medicine and Surgery (Macmillan, New York) for more details.

Although this subject does not strictly fall under the heading "orthopædic surgery," the author has introduced it more especially for his own students and assistants, as an aid to proper diagnostic technique and observation in orthopædic practice.

The X-rays, or Röntgen rays are produced by an electric discharge between two separated electrodes in a modified Crooke's or vacuum tube. They have the power of penetrating a large number of opaque objects; they affect a photographic plate and may be made visible to the eye also by means of a fluorescent screen known as a fluoroscope. There are thus three necessary parts to the X-ray outfit:

the tube, the electric exciting machine, and the receiving device, *i. e.*, the photographic plate, or fluoroscope.

The tube is a closed glass vessel or bulb in a high state of vacuum into which are hermetically sealed two metallic electrodes. These two electrodes are connected to the terminals of the exciting machine; the electrode connected to the positive terminal is called the anode, that to the negative the cathode. When the tube is in operation there is a stream of negatively charged particles issuing at a high velocity from the face of the cathode. This cathode stream has the peculiar property of exciting any body placed in its path in such a way that the body becomes the seat of the emanation known as the X-rays. Often the anode itself is used as this object, in which case the anode appears to be the source of the X-rays. In some tubes there is a special target for the purpose, but in either case the body emitting the X-ray is usually of sheet platinum or aluminum, turned in such a way as to throw the X-rays out through the side wall of the tube. The side walls themselves emit the X-rays throughout the region where they are struck by the cathode stream, as stray X-rays, but those opposite the center of the anodal target are the direct or primary X-rays and are more penetrative. This is at times availed of by having a tube of lead known as a focus tube or cylinder to "cut out" or absorb the stray emanations, between the X-ray tube and the part to be skiagraphed, insuring a clearer shadow.

The penetrative power of the rays depends in a large measure upon the degree of vacuum in the tube. The density of objects from a chemical standpoint depends on their atomic weight and it has been found that the X-rays penetrate those of low atomic weight easier than those of high atomic weight, which may be said in the human body to range from 1 for hydrogen to 40 for calcium.

In general there are two types of X-rays, rays of high penetration and rays of low penetration, and whenever a tube is in operation both types of ray are given off. It may be stated broadly, however, that the greater the degree of vacuum in the tube, *i. e.*, the "harder" to pass a current through the tube, or the "higher" its resistance, the greater the preponderance of the more highly penetrative rays over those of lower penetrative power, and vice versa. It is thus desirable to have some means for varying the degree of vacuum in a tube and for this purpose various self-regulating devices are provided. The most common form is the insertion, into a side bulb of the tube of a small quantity of some salt, which when heated by a flame or side spark, gives off a gas, thus lowering the vacuum. The operation of such a device is described more in detail below. A tube tends to become higher the more it is used.

For exciting the X-ray tube, a source of electricity at a very high difference of potential, or electromotive force is necessary; the higher the vacuum of the tube, the greater this difference of potential must be. Hence the exciting machine should have a range of e.m.f. corresponding to the working range of the tubes for various penetrating powers. It is also most desirable for the machine to have a range of variation of volume of output at any value of its e.m.f. or potential; thus, for instance, if it is giving a six-inch spark, it should be possible to vary the size of this spark from a thin to a voluminous or fat state. The time of exposure depends largely on this volume of discharge in the tube. Thus to secure definition of softer tissues a low vacuum should be used, and it is desirable that the exposure be short, for the more highly penetrative rays are always present to some degree, and a long exposure would enable these rays to obliterate the definition of the low rays. Thus if there is sufficient volume in the spark the exposure should be short and due only to the rays of lower penetrative power. High tubes and longer exposures are needed for bones and denser tissues.

EXCITING APPARATUS.

Three types of exciting machine are commonly used: (1) The Ruhmkorf induction coil; (2) the influence or static machine, *e. g.*, the Holtz or Wimshurst; (3) the alternating current transformer.

To secure the range of operation spoken of above, certain auxiliary apparatus is necessary in each case. In the case of the induction coil, the variation of the primary e.m.f. or difference of potential is one means, but besides this the interrupting device is also designed to vary the volume of discharge. Here we can only mention several forms and state that the author's observation of this class of apparatus inclines him to think the Wehnelt interrupter presents the greatest possibility of adaptation to variation of working range. Other interrupting devices are the electro-magnetic separate circuit break, and various forms of rotary direct breaks.

There are various types of influence machines on the market and the writer prefers the type named below.

The alternating current transformer has been used to some extent in places where direct current is not available. Results with this class of apparatus appear to be good in some cases, but it is open to the decided objection that it requires a special form of tube, and that the life of these tubes appears shorter (getting too high and becoming blackened) than those of the more common form. On the other hand the alternating current apparatus is much· simpler than either an induction coil or influence machine.

After five or six years' experience with a coil and subsequently six years' experience with a twenty-four plate Holtz-

Wimshurst static machine (Van Houten and Ten Broeck, New York), driven by a one-fourth horsepower electric motor the author is unhesitatingly in favor of the latter for constancy and reliability in results.

Much has been said and written about static machines not working on damp days and requiring a much longer exposure than the coils, but in the author's hands these claims have not been borne out and even if invariable these objections are more than counterbalanced by the annoyance of breakdowns in complicated coils and interrupters.

Suitable supports from the floor come with the various machines to hold the tubes at any desired angle.

It is not the province of this work to describe the details of an induction coil and break or a static machine, rheostat, and the motor run by an electric current, gas or water, but suffice it to say with a static machine, the necessary current can be as readily supplied to illuminate an X-ray tube, as one would turn on the current of an electric fan or other similar apparatus. When the static machine is developing sufficient energy (800,000 to 1,000,000 volts with an amperage of one half or less) it is usually at the maximum speed, needed for a very high tube.

TUBES.

The X-ray tube is preferably of the vacuum regulating variety, such as Queen & Co.'s, Philadelphia, or preferably the Edison Decorative and Miniature Lamp Co.'s, of Harrison, N. J., or Möller's German tubes, or Friedlander's. It is a matter of ease after a little experience to tell whether the light is of the desired degree of intensity for fluorescent examination or for photographic purposes. This degree of intensity of the light is regulated by the spark-gaps attached to the coil or static machine and by the vacuum regulator of the tube. This presupposes that a good tube is dealt with and it is preferable to purchase one of a high vacuum to start with. Various synonymous terms have been employed to describe tubes; namely "high" or "low" vacuum, "hard" or "soft" tubes and tubes of high resistance or low resistance, the last being the best terms as being measurable. If a tube has a vacuum of such an exhaustion that a very strong current is required to illuminate it, it is said to be of high resistance, hard or high vacuum. This degree of resistance can be measured by a spark gap introduced into the circuit of the tube by attaching one end of an insulated wire to one terminal of the tube already in circuit and moving the other end backward and forward from the other end of the tube. If the tube is of high resistance between the loose end of the testing wire and the far end of the tube a spark will jump for several inches, depending on the highness of the resistance in the tube. On the other hand, if the resistance is low, the tube will light up with but little electromotive force, which will pass through the tube in preference to jumping over the air space between the wires, even if this space is a small fraction of an inch or centimeter. Of course, this fraction depends on the lowness of the tube's resistance.

Nearly all modern tubes have three terminals, the anode into which the current passes from the positive terminal of the exciting machine, the cathode from which the current leaves the tube after the cathode rays have been reflected back on the target of the positive pole from which spring the X-rays and the third terminal which is usually a tube or bulb containing some salt, such as potassium hydroxide, easily converted into a gas when an electric current passes through and heats it. If a tube is too high the positive wire is attached to this third terminal and the current turned on for a few seconds thus driving the gas from the salt into the vacuum tube, until the vacuum is lowered the desired amount for the particular kind of work needed. The positive wire is then returned to the anodal terminal. We also have switches or detachable automatic vacuum regulators, such as the bario-vacuum regulator and automatic vacuum regulating tubes. · (Fig. 17.)

Williams made the valuable observation that very high vacuum tubes were better adapted to fluoroscopic work and the less high tubes to photography.

The character of the tube can be told by the fluoroscopic screen after the tube is lighted up in a darkened room; if very high, the hand when held between the light and the screen wlil

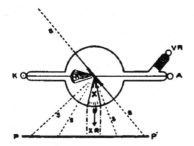

FIG. 17. X-RAY TUBE. *A*, ANODE. *K*. KATHODE. *KS*, KATHODE STREAM. *X*, X-RAYS. *XR*. PRIMARY X-RAYS. *S*, STRAY X-RAYS. *P—P'*, PHOTOGRAPHIC PLATE. *VR*, VACUUM REGULATING ATTACHMENT.

appear white with little or no contrast between the soft parts and the bone. If, on the other hand the whole hand appears black the tube is too low. A tube midway between a very high tube and a low one renders the bones rather black in contrast to the lighter soft parts and it is a tube of this character that gives the best results in X-ray photography. The very high tube is better for fluoroscopic observations and where extraordinary penetration is required in photography, such a case as the pelvis of a fat person. It is not necessary to keep a room dark for radiographic purposes after the character of the tube has been determined.

In order to study a case thoroughly and for diagnosis the radiograph will be found much more useful than the fluoroscope in orthopædic surgery.

PLATES.

The author has found the Cramer X-ray, Seed, Hammer & Stanley photographic plates the most useful and the sizes most frequently used are the 5 x 7, 8 x 10, 11 x 14 and 14 x 17 inches. In the photographic dark room they must be put in first a black and then an orange envelope before taking in the light for use in radiography. It is undesirable to buy the plates already in envelopes as they deteriorate when so packed for any time. The film side of the plate is to be put away from the flap side of the envelopes. The dark room where plates are kept should have a brick wall between it and the exciting machine, otherwise the unexposed plates may be affected by the powerful X-rays. If this is not practicable the stock of plates should be kept in a lead . covered or lined box.

SHADOWGRAPHY.

It is to be remembered that radiographs are shadow pictures and just as we know the shadow of an object cast by a candle is much clearer, the nearer the object is to the shadow, so in radiography the nearer the bone is to the photographic plate, the more sharp is the detail.

Further, the clearness, absence of distortion and magnification in the shadow depend on the distance of the light from the object and of the object from the surface on which the shadow falls. Also the rays of light must fall perpendicularly through the object on the receiving surface.

We are all familiar with the distorted shadows made on the wall in a lighted room as a person moves around in it at varying distances from the light and receiving surfaces.

So in radiography one cannot be too careful in order to obtain accurate results to have the vacuum tube at the proper distance from the photographic plate and the part to be skiagraphed. Also the rays from the tube which emerge in parallel lines must fall perpendicularly on the photographic plate with the long axis of the tube parallel to it and the center of the anode directly over the most important part to be skiagraphed. If the rays are falling vertically on the plate it can be determined in the following way: A square block of wood 4 x 4 inches has two nails driven partly into its perpendicular median line two inches apart, so that if a shadow is cast vertically down but one nail appears, the two shadows blending; thus, if viewed from below with the fluoroscope, one can tell by this device if the position of the anode is correct.

The distance of the tube from the plate should vary therefore with the thickness of the part and the distance of the contained bone to the plate, thus in the case of the hand, the tube should be from ten to twelve inches away from the plate and in skiagraphing the hip it should be from eighteen to thirty inches. The tube should never be closer to the skin than ten inches for fear of burning the patient and distorting the image by magnification, but many beginners think if they did not get a good picture with the tube twelve inches away, if they should put it three or four away success would be assured. This of course is erroneous. Frequently if the exposure is at all prolonged with the tube so close a serious dermatitis or burn is the result and from no other cause. In over ten years' experience the author has never had the misfortune of having such an accident with coil or static machine.

THE FLUOROSCOPE.

The fluoroscope is a pyramidal truncated pasteboard box, whose base is covered by a fluorescent screen and the apex has an opening to receive the eyes and exclude the light. It is covered with black cloth. The fluorescent screen of card board is covered with a layer of the tungstate of calcium or the platino-cyanide of barium. The first named is the more durable and satisfactory, but it should not phosphoresce after the X-ray light is out, as they sometimes do and should be tested for this defect in making a selection.

THE POSITION OF THE PATIENT.

The patient should be put in a convenient position and comfortably supported to insure immobility. After testing the apparatus to see that all is working properly and the part to be radiographed has been properly centered and placed under the anode of the vacuum tube at a proper distance, the photographic plate in its envelope is only then brought into the room and put into position and the tube lighted up. (The anode should be at an angle of 45° with the plate to properly reflect the cathode rays as X-rays.)

For the back, neck, shoulder, chest, abdomen, pelvis, hip joint, and for antero-posterior views of the thigh and leg the patient should lie flat on his back on a table with a folded blanket under him for comfort.

An ordinary table may be made by a carpenter 6 feet long, 2 feet wide, and 2 feet high; along one edge and each end a strip 2 inches wide $\frac{1}{8}$ of an inch thick is nailed and three similar strips crosswise at intervals of 17 inches apart. The whole can then be covered with oilcloth or heavy leather tightly, leaving one edge of the table open, however, so that photographic plates can be slipped under it into the compartments made by the strips, without disturbing the patient.

When it is desired to use a plate smaller than a 14 x 17, kits may be employed, as one would use a kit for a smaller photographic plate in a smaller plateholder. By passing a string or two around a plate on introducing it into one of these compartments it may be readily withdrawn after an exposure.

For the elbow, forearm and hand, an extension top table should be used to support the arm, while the patient sits in a chair.

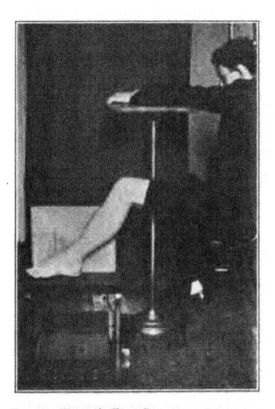

FIG. 18. WEIGEL'S FOOT STAND AND ARM STAND.

The small holes in the platform of the foot stand are for the reception of the X-ray tube holder in any desired position.

For the lateral views of the thigh, leg and knee joint a device should be at hand to support the leg and photographic plate at the same time while the patient is in a sitting posture, such as Weigel's knee support.

For lateral views of the foot and ankle with a medial surface in contact with the plate, there should be a footstool to support both plate and foot. (Such apparatus has been devised by Dr. L. A. Weigel, of Rochester, and can be had of Van Houten & Ten Broeck, New York). For antero-posterior views of the foot, the plate is put on the floor, the foot placed on it and thus the radiogram is made. (Figs. 18 and 19.)

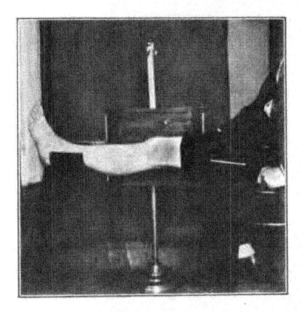

FIG. 19. WEIGEL'S KNEE STAND.

It is essential to success to secure immobilization and to have these comfortable supports to the various parts of the body, otherwise the negatives will have double lines with every slight movement of the patient and not be sharply defined. At times it may in addition be necessary to further immobilize the part by buckling webbing straps around the plate and part to be skiagraphed.

EXPOSURE.

With these details in mind we next come to the question of the length of time for exposure of the plate to the Röntgen light. This involves three points, the light producing power of the machine, the density of the part and the distance of the bony structure desired from the plate. Thus the hand can be radiographed in from 5 to 60 seconds, while the hip joint would require from 3 to 15 minutes, and the chest, although perhaps as thick as the hip, would require only half as long, being less dense. One reads in the journals of instantaneous radiography but the author has had no experience with it.

DEVELOPMENT OF THE PLATE.

Given a good X-ray apparatus, perhaps nothing counts for so much in success as proper development of the plate, which cannot be done hastily but only with painstaking care.

In all handling of these large plates, it is to be borne in mind that whether the plate is wet or dry, the fingers are to be kept off the sensitized film side. Whether in putting the plate in the non-actinic envelopes or in the early stages of development, it is to be kept as far from the bright rays of the red and yellow dark room lantern as is possible, to avoid fogging. The film side of the plate can be told some distance from the light by showing no reflection of the light as the glass side does, and this film side should be next to the smooth side of the envelope and *not* that with the flap. The film side of course is put next to the patient at the time of the exposure.

When the plate is taken into the dark room for development after the envelopes are removed the film side is thoroughly moistened under the water tap, so that when the chemicals come in contact with it, they will act uniformly all over its surface.

The plate is then put into a developing tray face up. These large trays are expensive but inexpensive trays can be made of wood and lined with rubber cloth.

The developing solution is then poured on. Any of the ready-for-use developers gotten in powder form may be used for simple diagnostic work and of these Carbutt's or Seed's metol-hydro powders will be found as useful for X-ray plates as they are for ordinary photographic negatives, positive films or bromide prints.

One powder is added to from four to eight ounces of water, depending on whether the exposure is long or short, respectively. The more dilute the solution the more detail will be brought out in the resulting negative but the longer will development take. More errors are made in the under-development of X-ray negatives than overdevelopment. Proper development before "fixing" requires from fifteen minutes to an hour and a half, depending on the amount of detail required; one should begin with a weak solution and then use a stronger.

Where detail, perfection and intensity in the negative are desired the following formula will be found one of the best:

Dr. L. A. Weigel's Formula.

(A) Stock solutions:
     Pyrogallic acid ʒi
     Alcohol fʒiv
     (developer)
(B) Potassium bromide
     (restrainer) 10% solution fʒiv
(C) Sodium sulphite crystals
     (clarifier) saturated solution Oij
(D) Sodium carbonate crystals.
     (accelerator) saturated solution Oij

To mix Dr. Weigel's solutions one to four drachms of (A) is added to one to four ounces of (C) and four to twelve ounces of water, depending on the size of the plate. This is poured on the moistened plate, which is then rocked backwards and forwards to insure the chemicals coming uniformly into contact with all parts of the plate.

After a few minutes one-half to two drachms of solution (B) is added and then one or two ounces of (D).

While constantly rocking the solutions over the plate, an ounce or more of the carbonate is added from time to time until the high lights become intensely black, the image gets a grayish dark hue and the outlines of the image appear on the under side, which also is grayish. Some fifteen to thirty or more minutes are required to complete development and the error is more frequently made of using too little carbonate towards the latter part of the process, adding little by little, than adding too much. From four to eight ounces of this accelerator is usually needed in this formula.

The pyrogallic acid formula given with the Cramer X-ray plates is a most excellent one also, and indeed simpler than Weigel's.

Many now prefer metol or similar developers to pyrogallic acid, but the latter in the long run gives much more beautiful results.

No matter what developing solution is used, the plate, when development is completed, is again washed under the tap and then put into the fixing bath until the plate is translucent and all the white of the silver albuminate has disappeared from it. This requires fifteen to twenty minutes more.

Formula of Fixing Bath.

Sodium hyposulphite ʒviii
Water   Oij

The acid fixing bath recommended with some plates may be used and is especially useful with all plates in summer for clearing, hardening and fixing. After the plate is thoroughly fixed, the glass side is washed under the tap to remove adherent chemicals and then placed film side up under the running water for fifteen or twenty minutes. Then the glass side is washed with the hand, being careful of the film on the reverse side. Finally it is turned up on edge and dried.

The interpretation of radiographs will be given under the diseases described.

THE X-RAY STEREOSCOPE.

A stereoscope is, as we all know, an instrument by means of which pictures or plane representations of objects possessing three dimensions are seen not as plane objects, but with an appearance of solidity or in relief as in the ordinary vision of the objects themselves.

The common stereoscope of the household by which we are accustomed to view photographs of Niagara and the like is known to physicists and opticians as the *refracting* stereoscope, as there are two refracting lenses in the eyepieces, which fuse the two pictures into one, showing depth. This form of stereoscope was invented by Sir David Brewster and presented by him to the Royal Society of Edinburgh in 1843 and 1844. These instruments were then made by Dubroscq, a Parisian optician, in 1849, at a time when Daguerre and Talbot were making their discoveries in photography, so that photographs which were taken by two cameras forming a certain definite angle to the object, could be used in the stereoscope instead of the careful drawings, which had been used up to that time by Sir Charles Wheatstone, the discoverer of binocular vision and the first and original *reflecting* stereoscope. As early as 1832, Newman, a philosophical instrument-maker, made a *reflecting* stereoscope for Sir Charles Wheatstone, but the latter did not publish his researches until 1838, when his paper on contributions to the "Physiology of Vision, Part the First" appeared in the Philosophical Transactions.

It is with this reflecting stereoscope of Wheatstone that we are especially interested in the examination of X-ray negatives.

The first instrument of this kind for this purpose was made in this country under the direction of Dr. L. A. Weigel, of Rochester, N. Y. Dr. Weigel has done more than perhaps any one man in this country to perfect the technique of radiography, especially as applied to orthopædic surgery, to correct errors of distortion and interpretation in skiagraphs and in the proper chemical development of X-ray negatives.

Now a word as to the principle of the Wheatstone stereoscope.

There are two mirrors with their backs towards each other forming an angle of 90°, where they are united. The nose is placed at the intersection of these two mirrors and each eye gazes at a reflection in its special mirror, so that if two calculatedly dissimilar pictures of the same object be placed in planes at 45° to and beyond the mirrors, the impression or recombination will be made in the mind that there is but one image and depth or the third dimension of space will be apparent also by the binocular phenomena, whatever that may be. (Fig. 20.)

The Weigel instrument, to use his language, consists of "a bed piece upon which, at its center, two mirrors inclined to each other at an angle of 90° are mounted on a slide, having a forward and backward movement to facilitate adjustment. At the angle formed by the mirrors, a screen with openings for the eyes is placed.

"Two grooved frames, for holding the negatives, face the mirrors at 45° and are adjustable by a simple sliding motion in two directions, one at right angles to the base and the other parallel with it. In the base of these frames there is

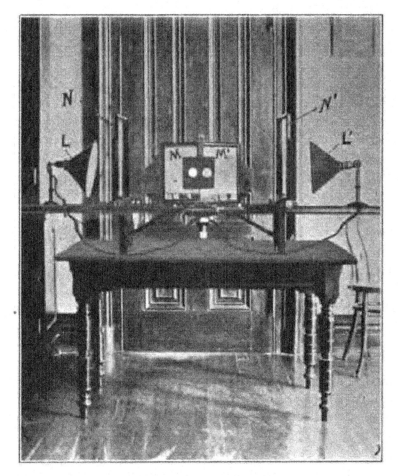

FIG. 20. WEIGEL'S X-RAY STEREOSCOPE. *L*, LIGHT. *M*, MIRROR. *N*, NEGATIVE.

also a mechanism controlled by a milled head screw, for vertical adjustment. By means of these various movements the images of the two negatives reflected in the mirrors may be quickly adjusted until they are accurately superimposed and the stereoscopic relief is obtained. Transillumination of the negatives is necessary and this is best secured by artificial light. The most convenient and satisfactory source of illumination is from electric lights. In my apparatus a sixteen candlepower lamp is placed behind each negative. Flexible conducting cords from these lamps are wired in parallel to a single keysocket attached to the under side of the bed. An electric light cord of convenient length and having an extension plug at each end is used to connect the apparatus with any available lamp socket in the room. One of the plugs is placed in the keysocket of the apparatus and the other attached to the source of the illumination selected. For concentrating the light on the negatives, an ordinary metal shade or reflector surrounds the electric light bulb, which should preferably be of ground glass. An even diffusion of the light is still further secured by having one side of the negative frames covered with a sheet of ground celluloid, which is lighter and less fragile than ground glass. The lamp brackets are adjustable vertically, and as they are attached to an independent base, the distance between the light and the negatives may easily be regulated, according to the varying density of the plates. Where an electric light plant is not available, Welsbach gas lamps or acetylene bicycle lamps may be substituted for the illumination.

"The negative holders are square and large enough to take in plates of all sizes up to and including 11 x 14 inches, and may be placed in the frames either vertically or horizontally. For the smaller sized plates it is advisable to use masks of black press board or other material to cut off all extraneous light.

"Although this apparatus is somewhat large, the bedpiece being six feet long, it may be stored in any ordinary closet, as all the movable parts are detachable. The mirrors are fastened to the slide by thumbscrews and are so hinged as to fold upon themselves when removed from the apparatus. The negative frames, lampbrackets, eyescreen, keysocket, etc., are also readily detached, leaving nothing but the bedpiece with the legs, and, as the latter are hinged and fold against the under side of the bed, very little space is required for it. The apparatus may be set up complete for use in less than five minutes."[11]

The value of this instrument lies chiefly in the examination of the direction of fractures, of dislocations and their components, the location of foreign bodies, whether on the right, left, anterior or posterior aspect of a bone, the direction of piercing foreign bodies, such as needles, nails, bullets, etc., none of which are shown in a flat negative nor the positive obtained from it. The location and depth of tubercular foci prior to erasion, foreign or loose bodies in joints, etc., can be usefully examined by this method.

Thus, for example, also a Pott's fracture of the fibula of the right leg might in the ordinary negative give one the impression that the fragments were in apposition, whereas if viewed in the stereoscope we might see that the lower fragment was half an inch or more external or internal to the the upper fragment; union would therefore be delayed or be imperfect, if not detected.

So in negatives or prints of foreign bodies, such as needles or pins in the hands or feet, which are so deceptive in every way at times, we can see whether they have "migrated," as the expression goes, to the palmer or plantar aspect or the reverse; which is the larger end of the needle and the obliquity of its entrance to the soft parts, etc.

It may be argued that this is a great deal of trouble for a very small matter, but in reply to this it may be said in

[11] L. A. Weigel: N. Y. Med. Jour., Nov. 16, 1901.

regard to fractures or dislocations in an important case or one in which a possible suit for damages may result, it is not a small matter.   In regard to time and trouble it is but a question, of perhaps from a few seconds to a few minutes more in making two negatives, instead of one, in regard to the hand or arm and from two to five minutes in regard to the foot or leg.   The question of additional time to the development will add perhaps thirty minutes for the additional negative, unless one is equipped with those most useful adjuncts of the dark room, a double pan, to develop two at once, thus also effecting uniform development in two similar negatives.

STEREOSCOPIC X-RAY NEGATIVES.

One more word in regard to making these two negatives, which for stereoscopic purposes, should be dissimilar views of the same object but of a calculated dissimilarity.

For example, if we are taking a profile view of the knee we should locate our Crooke's tube on a line say 12 to 18 inches from the patient, a safe distance, and the center of this line should be opposite the center of the joint; now for the first negative the anode of the tube should be approximately $1\frac{1}{2}$ to 2 inches to the right of this center and the exposure made.   For the second negative the tube must be moved $1\frac{1}{2}$ to 2 inches, as the case may be, to the left of this center and the second exposure made.   This gives what we might call the proper inclination of the optic (or Crooke's tube) axes.   Of course, the greater the distance of the Crooke's tube from the body the greater must be the distance we move the anode for each exposure.

CHAPTER IV.

THE PATHOGENESIS OF DEFORMITY.

WOLFF'S LAW AND ITS COROLLARIES.

If one attempts to analyze the ætiology of the various deformities seen, one will find that they may be classed as those that are congenital in origin, those that are due to trauma, osseous, periosteal or articular disease, post-paralytic contracture, atrophy or weakness, those resulting from habit or burns, and finally those in which faulty nutrition or attitude are to blame.[12]

If one looks further back for the ætiology of acquired deformity one finds two theories; one, the older, known as the Volkmann-Hueter or "pressure-atrophy theory,"[13] and the other, the theory of Julius Wolff, of Berlin, known as the "functional transformation of bone" or "the functional pathogenesis of deformity."[14]

Both theories possess points which claim acceptance, but on the whole that of Wolff, though but little emphasized or even mentioned in many treatises on orthopædic surgery, deserves the wider scientific recognition.

The Volkmann-Hueter theory claims that "consequent upon muscular weakness that faulty attitude is assumed, in

---

[12] R. T. Taylor: American Journal of Medical Sciences, Dec., 1902; Trans., American Orthopædic Association, vol. xv, 1902.

[13] Volkmann v. Pitha u. Billroth's Chirurgie, ii, Abth. ii, p. 629, *et seq.;* Hueter: Virchow's Archiv., xxv, p. 572, *et seq.*

[14] Wolff: Gesetz. d. Transformation d. Knochen, Berlin, 1892; Berlin klin. Wochenschr., 1900, no. 18; Archiv f. klin. Chir., Band liii, Heft 4; Ueber d. Wechselbeziehungen zw. d. Form. u. d. Function d. einzelmen Gebide d. organisms, Leipzig, 1901.

consequence of which one side of a joint (or of the trunk) is subjected to greater pressure than is normal and the opposite side sustains less pressure than is normal. Assuming that during growth the normal development of the joint depends upon the maintenance of normal conditions of intra-articular pressure, it was explained that the increased pressure on the concave side interfered with the normal growth of the bone, or even caused atrophy of the bony tissue already formed, while on the convex side the subnormal pressure permitted an overgrowth of bone."[15] For example, if this is applied to knock-knee, a manifestation of rickets, one is naturally led to believe that the internal condyle of the femur shows an overgrowth and the external an atrophy, but Mikulicz,[16] Macewen,[17] Blanchard,[18] and others, have shown that these changes in the articular surfaces and the epiphyses are not constantly present in knock-knee, but that the principal deformity exists in the diaphyses or shafts of the femur and tibia, which most authors, even today continue to overlook and still describe the pathogenesis of this affection in conformity with the Volkmann-Heuter theory.

The followers of this theory applied the same reasoning to the changes produced in the vertebral bodies in lateral curvature of the spine, in which the shape is changed from a quadrilateral to a wedge shape by the "superincumbent weight," producing pressure atrophy on the concave side of the spinal curve and hypertrophy on the convex.

This reasoning, although natural and at first sight reasonable, is not substantiated by anatomical, pathological and mathematical demonstration (the last named, however, partially) as will be seen from Wolff's researches and able exposition of the subject.

[15] Freiberg: Transactions of the Amer. Orthopæd. Assoc., vol. xv, 1902.
[16] Arch. f. Klin. Chir., xxiii, p. 561.
[17] Lancet, September, 1884.
[18] Amer. Journ. Orthoped. Surg., vol. i, no. 1.

Wolff's Law, to quote Freiberg again, is as follows:

"Every change in the form and function of the bones, or of their function alone, is followed by certain definite changes in their internal architecture and equally definite secondary alterations of their external conformation, in accordance with mathematical laws."

Wolff formulated his law after painstaking study of the various bones of the body under normal and abnormal conditions, each as a whole or in sections, comparing the cortex and the spongy portion with the functional demands on each, and concluded that the cortical layer was simply a condensation of the spongiosa to meet the demands placed upon it. He attached great importance to the resemblance between the trabecular arrangement in a frontal section of the femur and Cullmann's mathematical drawing of a Fairbairn crane, first insisted upon by Van Meyer, in which the trajectories necessary to support a load of thirty kilogrammes, approximately the weight of an adult, gave a picture practically identical with the internal arrangement of the trabeculæ and lamellæ in the human femur deprived of its trochanters. The consolidation of the trajectories on the surface would constitute the cortex as compared with the bone. (Fig. 21.)

Of course such a calculated mathematical drawing, to have a perfect and absolute similarity to the femur, would of necessity have to include not only the demands to be put upon it in the upright position, but in every other possible position which it might assume, and the various pressures, stresses, and shearing strains to which it must be subjected by the muscles.

Such a drawing must show what part the trochanters play as their trabeculæ are found continuous with those of the shaft and neck, and their portion in functional burden bearing is no small one, and the drawing must be based on a standard quality of bone, when the "factor of safety" enters into the consideration, as an engineer would calculate the quality of the steel in making the specifications for any structure.

Thus it will be seen that such a calculation to produce a mathematical drawing by graphic statics of the osseous structure would involve the greatest amount of intelligence, knowledge and time and even then would be well-nigh impossible. Nevertheless the resemblance of Cullmann's

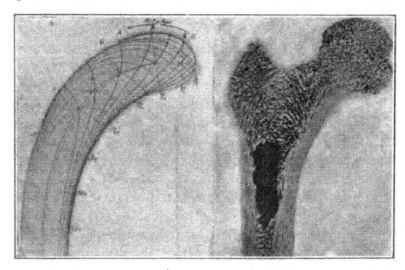

FIG. 21. FAIRBAIRN CRANE AND FEMUR.   (Freiberg.)

Fairbairn crane may be regarded as very suggestive and remarkable.

Working from this, Wolff found that the external form and internal architecture was dependent on the function demanded of the bone and that the external contour and internal architecture always correspond exactly, the former representing mathematically the last curve uniting the various trajectories (lamellæ) which make up the internal structure (spongiosa.) The compact substance is to be regarded simply as a condensation of the spongiosa. This covers his first corollary that "external shape and internal architecture are dependent on function solely."

From the theory of the "functional shape" it is an easy step to that of the "functional pathogensis of deformity" his second corollary. If the internal structure and external contour correspond exactly to their demands and if they represent an adaptation to normal function only, then an alteration in the static demands made upon the bones must be followed by the proper transformation in structure, both internal and external, and as the result of these we have the gradual deformity in the "narrower sense," as distinguished from sudden deformity caused by trauma, bone disease, etc., which Wolff speaks of as deformity in the "broader sense."

Thus deformity is to be regarded as a physiological adaptation of the structure to pathological static requirements, therefore to "pathological function." Or we could express it that, pathological function produces a physiological bone transformation to meet new static demands.

The great value of Wolff's research is borne out conclusively by anatomical and pathological findings, and the author has deemed it of sufficient importance to go into the subject thus briefly to correct in the minds of his readers preconceived ideas of the older theory of atrophy and hypertrophy in bone according to the Volkmann-Hueter theory.

Viewing the example cited of knock-knees from Wolff's standpoint, it will be found on section that instead of an atrophy of the external condyle there has been a bone transformation and condensation or osteosclerosis and the internal condyle has not hypertrophied, but undergone an osteoporosis, as the greater strength and weight-bearing in such a case falls on the outer side of the bone. In fact, the cortex above and below the knee will be found thicker on the outer side, to withstand greater strain, than the inner,

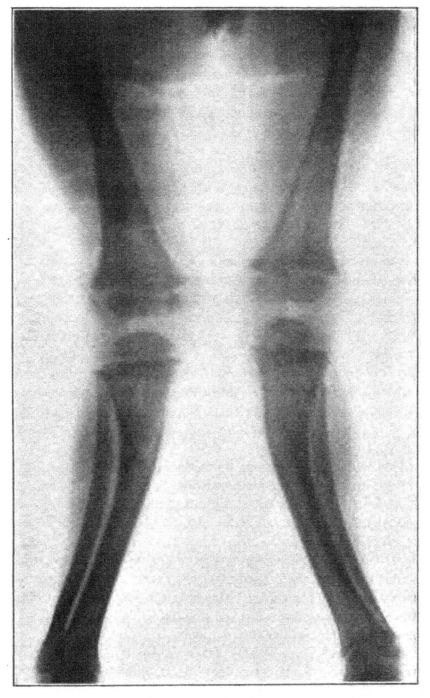

FIG. 22.   KNOCK-KNEE X-RAY.

Attention is especially called to the thickened cortex on the concave side of the
bones.

whereas we know that in the normal bones the cortex is approximately equal on the external and medial sides in a transverse section. (Fig. 22.)

One so often hears explanations advanced, chiefly by parents, as to why a child is bandy-legged, on the ground that the child is so heavy; one is therefore apt to fall into the error that the superincumbent weight is entirely responsible for the deformity and not the physiological bone transformation to meet faulty or pathological static habits.

Wolff's law is most important of application in the treatment of various orthopædic affections and especially in the post-operative treatment of them, to allow sufficient time to elapse for this bone transformation in the direction of normal or a reversal of the pathological transformation, which has resulted in the deformity. Thus, for example, many surgeons unfamiliar with orthopædic measures are surprised to find a club-foot that has been operated on by division of the contracted tendons relapse, when the foot had not been held by a suitable apparatus, not only to prevent a recontraction of the soft parts, but also to *permit of bone adaptation* (i. e., functional transformation) to the changed condition.

This law also helps us to understand why it is important in certain conditions, such as knock-knee and bowlegs, to overcorrect the deformity in treatment, so that, what we may speak of as an osseous balance may be obtained. Thus in lateral curvature of the spine, if it were possible to hold the trunk for a sufficiently long period twisted in a direction diametrically opposed to that of the deformity, it might be reasonable to suppose that the resultant mean of the two curves would approximate the normal. This will be dwelt upon more at length under scoliosis.

The application of Wolff's law will be referred to from time to time in considering the other different diseases.

For purposes of classification we will consider the deformities in the following manner, as far as possible:

1. Those deformities due to tuberculous disease of the bone.

2. Those deformities due to non-tuberculous disease of the bone.

3. Those deformities due to congenital malformations.

4. Those deformities due to paralytic affections or weakness.

5. Those deformities due to faulty nutrition of the bones.

6. Those deformities due to trauma, burns, etc.

CHAPTER V.

TUBERCULAR LESIONS OF THE SPINE.

POTT'S DISEASE.

Pott's disease is a pathological process of tubercular origin which attacks the bodies of one or more adjacent vertebræ.

Synonyms. Humpback, hunchback; caries of the spine; tuberculous osteitis of the vertebræ; angular curvature; antero-posterior spinal curvature; spinal curvature; spondylitis and kyphosis. Of these, by far the most preferable are tuberculous osteitis of the vertebræ and kyphosis, which indicate the exact nature of the trouble; kyphosis meaning a backward curvature. Lordosis means a spinal curvature forward and scoliosis means a lateral spinal curvature.

HISTORICAL NOTES.

This disease was mentioned as far back as B. C. 783 by Galen and Hippocrates in their writings, and they speak of it as "tubercle within and without the lungs." Ambroise Paré wrote of it and used a brass cuirass to treat it in 1590.

Sir Percival Pott, of London, in 1779 gave first an accurate description of the gross lesions of the disease in his work, entitled "Remarks on that Kind of Palsy Affecting the Lower Limbs in Curvature of the Spine," therefore, since his time, it has borne his name.

The disease is not limited to the Anglo-Saxon, European, African or Asiatic races, but it existed in the prehistoric American, as is shown by the specimen of an Indian skeleton in the Peabody Museum at Cambridge, Mass.

PATHOLOGY.

A small spot of hyperæmia of gray or grayish red granulations is first seen usually in the anterior spongy portion of the bodies of the vertebræ due to the irritation of the bacillus tuberculosis finding a favorable seat for growth in a point of lowered vitality; these granulomatous areas are found to contain characteristic gray or yellow tubercles, which are composed of one or more giant cells having several nuclei and around them massed epitheloid cells, which in turn are surrounded by lymphoid cells. Scattered through this tubercle may be seen, in properly stained preparations, the bacillus of tuberculosis of Koch, either in the giant cells or between them and the lymphoid cells usually. The infection in the majority of cases comes to the bones by way of the blood or possibly lymphatics or by contiguity with other tuberculous tissue.

This spot becomes larger and redder, the center becomes opaque and grayish with a zone around it of hyperæmic granulation tissue. The process causing this gray spot is known as "caseation," and is produced possibly by the toxine of the bacilli and the massing together of the cells around the tubercle, and causing the fatty and cheesy degeneration and necrosis of the central part of the tubercle. Lacunar resorption of the bone always occurs at the seat of the tuberculous granulations and the bone trabeculæ become necrotic. If the process is rapid the caseous node thus formed contains these necrotic trabeculæ, which in a slow process are absorbed entirely. The hyperæmic zone is the area of tubercular granulation tissue and once started increases by peripheral extension. During the later and reparative stages of this process this area becomes less vascular and is converted into dense fibrous tissue.

The grayish area grows larger and becomes yellowish in color. As a result, we may have, not only as just mentioned, (*a*) caseation simply which is known as "caries sicca," in small nodes which advance slowly, but we may have (*b*) caseation with suppuration, which last is known as "caries necrotica" with liquefaction into tuberculous "pus," so-called, to form "cold abscesses," in which swelling is the only inflammatory sign present, redness, heat and pain being absent. As a result of this suppuration, we naturally have abscesses formed of broken down bone tissue and tubercles, which (1) may either point in various directions, discharge and form sinuses; or (2) the masses of caseous material, or the purulent collection may become incapsulated by the surrounding fibrinous and inflammatory tissue, "the so-called granulation tissue," and in turn be absorbed or calcified. (*c*) In either "caries sicca" or "caries necrotica," we may have the process extend by the blending with other granulo-matous areas or the actual extension of the original process, from the multiplication of the bacilli and the peripheral bone rarefaction and infection. This explains the putty-like nodes or nodules containing cheesy or calcareous material found in hard bone, and constitute the tubercular bone abscess, hence the name, "tubercular osteitis of the verte-bræ." These nodes may be from the size of a pea to that of a hazelnut. The liquefaction of these caseous masses result in a cloaca or cavity, or, as it is sometimes called, a cavernous excavation in the bone. In the osseous detritus one may find gritty remains of necrotic trabeculæ or even splinter-like fragments, which when large may deserve the name sequestra but these are not the rule. (Fig. 23.)

The transverse, articular and spinous processes are rarely affected as they are covered with hard bone, while the bodies are composed of more spongy bone, which are attacked usually in their anterior portions, softened and disinte-grated. As the disease extends to the periphery of one vertebral body, the contiguous surfaces of the adjacent vertebræ and intervertebral discs become involved in the tuberculous process. Some hold that the intervertebral cartilages are first involved; this may be so, but it is certainly not the rule. In any case, where the disease is of any extent, the intervertebral cartilages are absorbed only at the point of the disease. It is not an articular disease, however.

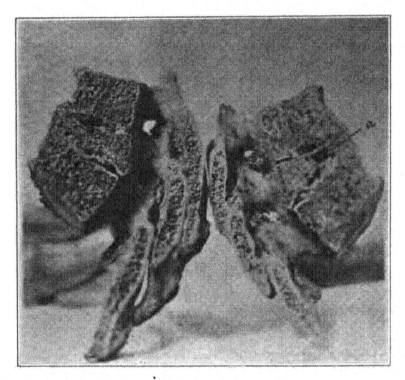

FIG. 23. SAGITTAL SECTION OF A CARIOUS VERTEBRAL BODY, SHOWING ABSCESS CAVITY AT *a*. (Courtesy of Dr. Holmes Smith.)

Primary disease at two points not adjacent is rare, though reported. (Fig. 24.) Superficial osteitis, not causing deformity and absorption of the intervertebral discs, is also rare.

Pus formation may be characteristic of certain cases and is usually indicative either of extensive disease or of an active process or possibly in certain cases to secondary infection with pyogenic cocci. Pus naturally gravitates downward, hence the frequency of psoas abscess in lower spinal caries. An abscess may point into the pharynx as a post-pharyngeal abscess, into the neck, back, axilla, lungs, abdomen, groin, etc., depending on the situation of the lesion and the line of least resistance. The abscess in the bone we may speak of as primary and that without it as secondary or consecutive. A primary abscess may be absorbed and a secondary abscess also, but the latter usually ruptures either outwards on the surface of the body or into some internal

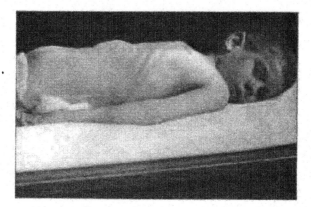

FIG. 24. CASE OF DOUBLE POTT'S DISEASE (DORSAL AND LUMBAR).

part and so form fistulous tracts or sinuses. At times the luxuriant growth of granulation tissue projects like a mushroom from the mouth of the sinus.

Pachy-meningitis and myelitis may complicate Pott's disease, not, however, from bone pressure, as the lumen of the spinal canal is not often narrowed; for example, deformity may increase and the paralysis may improve, or we may find paralysis without deformity. Usually paralysis comes from (1) external tuberculous pachy-meningitis by extension from the diseased bone to the external layer of the dura, which causes a myelitis by pressure at the point of the caries in the bone. The symptoms produced by this lesion are easy to understand, as the pressure is on the antero-lateral aspects of the spinal cord, and therefore the paralysis in the majority of cases will be a paralysis of motion. The myelitis is worse at the point of the meningitis and may destroy the cord there, or be a simple infiltration. Myelitis may be unilateral or bilateral and may extend up or down as an "ascending" or "descending" degeneration, but is usually localized at the area of disease of the bone. Secondarily, by pressure the myelitis causes a paralysis, which depends in extent entirely on the point and degree of the bone lesion. Occasionally paralysis is caused by œdema of the cord from the granulation tissue around the tuberculous area of the bone. In recovery, there is more or less sclerosis. As a rule the medullary surface of the dura is normal. We may (2) have a bone pressure myelitis from the dislocation of one of the vertebræ or separation of a posterior part of a verte-bral body into the spinal canal as a sequestrum, but this is extremely rare, and (3) we may have a myelitis from pres-sure of an abscess on the cord, due to its bursting into the vertebral canal. The cord is rarely, if ever, involved in the carious process and the postero-lateral aspect of it, is only involved in very severe cases, thus causing sensory as well as motor paralysis.

MORBID ANATOMY.

The morbid anatomy, of course, depends on the region of the spine involved, the extent and the duration of the disease.

In the dorsal region, the shape and capacity of the chest may be markedly and gradually changed in untreated cases on account of the softening of the bodies of the diseased vertebræ; the weight of the head and shoulders, pressing down from above, causes a backward projection of the spinous processes (corresponding to the diseased vertebræ) until two sound vertebral bodies resist further extension of the disease and healing, fibrous or bony ankylosis ensue. It is easy to understand from this that if the disease is extensive, that the direction of the ribs will be altered and in severe cases some will project downward, some horizontally and some will sink into the pelvis. (Fig. 25.) As the spine is shortened from above downward, so is the thorax; com-

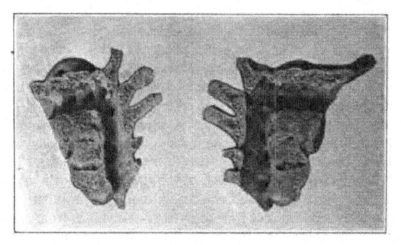

FIG. 25. RECTANGULAR DEFORMITY OF POTT'S DISEASE.
Attention is called to the fact that the spinal canal is not narrowed at the point of flexure.
(Courtesy of Dr. Holmes Smith.)

pensation in space for the thoracic viscera occurs by the bulging forward of the sternum, so that the antero-posterior diameter of the chest in a badly humpbacked person is longer than the transverse. In the cervical region the neck is shortened and the chin elevated; in the lumbar region the patient is shortwaisted and swaybacked.

On account of the intimate relationship which exists between the thoracic and abdominal aorta and the spinal column, when we have an antero-posterior bending of the spine, we may have the same flexion in the aorta, which in a bad case may produce a stenosis. This stenosis may cause hypertrophy of the heart and valvular lesions Cases have been reported of mitral incompetency and degeneration of the cardiac muscle walls. (Fig. 26.)

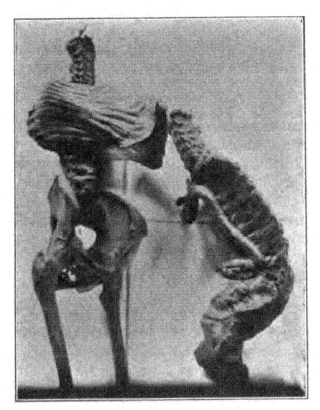

FIG. 26. SEVERE CASE OF POTT'S DISEASE AND FLEXURE OF AORTA.
(Museum of the University of Maryland.)

We may have phthisis pulmonalis, pleurisy or pericarditis due to extension from the carious bone, or improper and poor expansion of the lungs.

RECOVERY.

Recovery may occur without deformity at an early stage by incapsulation and cicatrization of the lesion and later by ankylosis of the bodies of the vertebræ with extreme deformity in untreated cases; this is, at best, an exceedingly slow process.

Recovery may occur by means of the granulation tissue, which in healing becomes less vascular and densely fibrous; or a formative osteitis may occur around the transverse and articular processes, which is the manner of recovery, that is the most usual under treatment and to be desired.

OCCURRENCE.

Sex plays but a minor part, although there are a few more males than females that have this disease.

Age. Childhood is much the most common time for this disease to develop, the majority of cases which will be seen, begin in children from five to fifteen years old. The youngest case that has been reported is one at eight weeks and the oldest at seventy-seven years.

Of all the cases of tubercular bone disease, that we see, about 26 per cent are spinal.

ÆTIOLOGY.

Pressure and Position. The erect attitude increases the superincumbent weight and further irritates any trauma and diseased focus that may exist in the bodies of the spinal vertebræ. It is not surprising, therefore, that this disease has not been reported in quadrupeds and is a penalty that the human race pays for walking erect.

LOCALIZATION OF DISEASE.

It is needless to say that this tubercular disease may involve the bodies of any of the vertebræ, but it is more common in certain regions than in others; the statistics from autopsies give us approximately the following relative proportions, as to the location of the tubercular focus; in the cervical region, 14 per cent; in the dorsal region 50 per cent; in the lumbar region 35 per cent; and the sacral region 1 per cent. Thus it will be seen that the disease is far more common in the dorsal region than in any of the others, and this has been attributed to the fact that the dorsal region is more exposed to injury, and furthermore in this region the normal spine is convex posteriorly, while in the cervical and lumbar regions it is concave posteriorly. In addition to this we will find that the center of gravity of the body passes through the cervical region, anterior to the dorsal region and through the lumbar region. As the ribs are attached to the dorsal vertebræ, if any diseased process exists in this region, every respiration that moves the ribs will inflict additional traumatism on the adjacent diseased focus.

PREDISPOSING CAUSES.

(a) Injuries of various kinds, such as falls, blows, and the like, are given in about 50 per cent of the histories as the predisposing cause of the disease. These produce an area of least resistance for the bacilli to grow upon, as a certain amount of stasis in the circulation exists at the seat of the contusion where the bacilli circulating in the blood or lymphatics find lodgment. This constitutes the infection atrium and after a slight injury it may be months before any symptoms of disease appear while the tubercles are developing and coalescing. Notwithstanding this slow development of the deformity the laity still think humpback is a "broken back" produced suddenly from an injury.

(b) Pressure from one cause or another, notably the superincumbent weight of the head, shoulders, etc., increase the curvature when once started.

(c) Lowered vitality, from some of the acute exanthemata of childhood, especially whooping cough, gives the system less resistance to the tuberculous invasion.

The exciting cause is the bacillus tuberculosis, causing caries of the vertebral body or bodies. This bone tuberculosis may be hereditary or acquired. Approximately 75 per cent of all the cases seen give an inherited family history of one form or another of tuberculosis. This is now thought to be by subsequent infection and not by direct intrauterine transmission from parent to child.

SYMPTOMS.

1. *Onset.*

All symptoms come on most gradually and the insidious onset of this disease is most characteristic.

2. *Muscular Rigidity.*

This is a constant and reliable, early and late symptom of practically all tubercular bone diseases, and in the spine, we will find it shown by the attitude, carriage and motions of the patient. Arbitrarily, we may divide the spine into four regions, in order to analyze these attitudes, etc., should disease attack any one of them.

The first region consists of the first three cervical vertebræ. (Whitman includes in this region the occipito-atloid articulation with its motions of flexion and extension.)

The second region consists of the fourth, fifth and sixth cervical vertebræ.

The third region extends from the seventh cervical through the tenth dorsal, and the last region extends from the eleventh dorsal through the fifth lumbar.

Now, if we examine the spine, we will find that in the first region, the normal motions of the vertebræ on each other, are those of rotation so that if any reflex stimulus, as seen in the acute stages of Pott's Disease, is given to the muscles, which regulate the motions in this region, we will find the head held in some position of torticollis or wryneck, therefore if we have a tubercular focus in this region, the child's head will be markedly rotated; all the muscles that are attached to this region will be rigidly contracted, and the

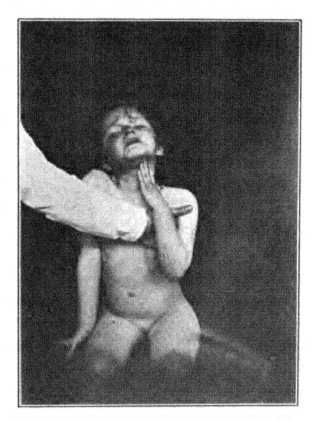

FIG. 27. ATTITUDE IN ACUTE CERVICAL DISEASE.

child will endeavor in every possible way to protect the injured part from jar or motion, as well as pressure. It will endeavor to remove the pressure by resting its head in its mother's lap or throwing itself across a table or chair, or by supporting the head with the hands. (Fig. 27.)

In the second region, we find that the vertebræ by their shape so articulate as to enable the head to be moved in flexion and extension, therefore in this region "the neuro-muscular expression" of the disease is that either the head of the child will be flexed forward with the chin resting on

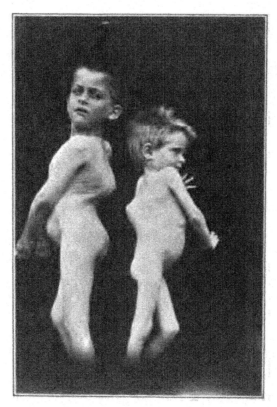

FIG. 28. TYPES OF MARKED DORSAL DISEASE.

the sternum or extended backward with the occiput resting on the spine. The child exerts the same precautions to protect the disabled part from injury, etc., as in cases in which the disease is in the first region. (Fig. 28.)

In the third region, the shoulders will be very squarely held and lifted up. The child will endeavor to prevent the upper part of the body, pressing on the diseased area and will support it by resting the hands on the knees instead of standing erect.   If asked to walk, it will do so by catching hold of chairs and tables in passing, to relieve the weakened spine of some of its burden.   Every motion is taken with

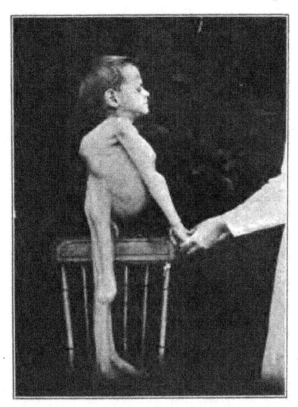

FIG. 29.   EXTREME DEFORMITY IN DORSAL DISEASE.

the greatest care to prevent jar and if any object is thrown on the floor and the child is requested to pick it up, it will do so by squatting instead of flexing the body forward, which procedure would jam the bodies of the adjacent well vertebræ against the diseased tender one.   (Fig. 32.)   In the same way, if a child with the disease in this region is put in a sitting posture with the legs extended on the examining table, it will be found that, unlike a normal child, it is unable to touch both feet with both hands at once, as it is unable to flex the spine forward owing to the muscular rigidity, which is Nature's method of protecting the diseased area. Also if such a child be placed on his hands and feet, and the examiner place the palms of his hands under his abdomen and lift him, the spine will be held straight and not bowed as is normal, for the same reason.

In the fourth region, as we have seen on examining the normal vertebræ of the spinal column, the convexity is forward, unlike the third region and at the greatest possible advantage for throwing the weight off of the diseased area, so that instead of the superincumbent weight of the body being anterior or on the diseased bodies of the vertebræ, it can be thrown posterior to them and supported on the articular and transverse processes of the lumbar region; thus, we will find the attitude in this region that of lordosis or sway-back, such children having almost a military bearing, but walking and moving with the greatest care, their stooping attitudes and motions are the same as those seen in the dorsal region. Such are the characteristics of active motions in the acute periods of this disease, especially in flexion of the spine before or after deformity has occurred. (Fig. 30.)

If such a case be placed face downward on an examining table and then so lifted by both legs at once, so that the sternum and face are still in contact with the table, it will be found in thus extending the spine that the vertebral column does not form an arc, as is normal, but is held straight and stiff by muscular spasm, not as though it were composed of many segments but as if it were one piece. (Fig. 38.)

In diseases in the lower dorsal and lumbar spine, we find reflex irritation of the psoas magnus muscle in some cases during the acute stage from its proximity with the diseased bodies, which produces the contraction, causing flexion of the thigh on the body; this is known as psoas contraction, and if it continues for a long time, so that the muscle and Y-ligament become shortened permanently, it

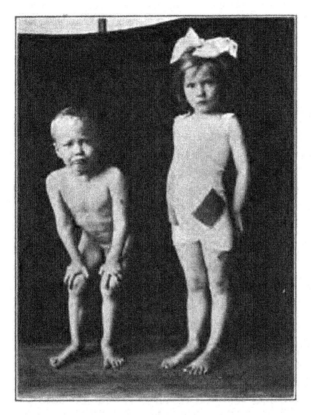

FIG. 30. POSTURES IN ACUTE DORSAL AND LUMBAR DISEASE.

may result in a very difficult deformity to overcome. There may be more or less flexion of the knees in all cases of Pott's Disease, owing to an effort on the part of the sufferer to lessen the shock on the diseased spine and make the step more elastic and as little on the heels as possible.

3. *Pain.*

Pain is a common symptom of Pott's Disease, but this pain is not usually present in the spinal region and is referred to the anterior portion of the body at the peripheral ends of the sensory nerves only when the disease is in the acute stage. This is due to pressure or inflammatory irritation of the nerves as they make their exit through the spinal foramina. In cervical Pott's Disease we will find the pain in the back of the head, or in the front of the neck or shoulders, while in dorsal disease the pain is in the front of the chest or stomach; and in lumbar disease the pain may be felt in the legs or hypogastric region or loins. It may simulate the pain of pharyngitis, pleurisy, pneumonia, peritonitis, cystitis, gastritis, etc. Careful examination of the spine is frequently necessary to make a diagnosis when pain exists without deformity. The pain as a rule is subacute, rarely being acute except when the disease is at its height. In cervical disease the reflex nerve irritation may give rise to a croupy cough and respiration like that present in laryngeal stenosis.

4. *Night Cries.*

The "night cry" is a symptom which indicates very active disease. They are heard in the early part of the night and are probably due to a relaxation of the muscular spasm and the grinding of the healthy bones against a diseased one. A child will give a sharp cry and by the time a parent or nurse has reached its side, it will be asleep again, the muscular spasm being reëstablished. This may be repeated several times. Patients that are old enough to describe their sensations say that the pain occasioned is of a dull, aching character and may persist for a little while. There is no dream with these night cries, as is the case in nightmare. Often the child does not really wake at all, is simply disturbed in its sleep and gives the cry.

5. *Deformity.*

Deformity is present after the disease has advanced and caused more or less destruction of the bodies of the vertebræ. It is easily made out by examining the spinous processes and may be extremely slight, constituting simply a small knuckle, or it may be extensive, including the spinous and transverse processes of several vertebræ with their ribs and produce a large hump. If one examines the spines carefully and notes the seventh cervical vertebra, the vertebra prominens, it is easy to see that normally there is no such projection in the others, so that even in slight disease, any such deformity is easily made out. This when present constitutes an antero-posterior deformity with the convexity backward. Occasionally we may see a lateral deviation, due to the diseased process being more extensive on one side of a vertebral body than on the other. As the vertebral bodies soften more and more from disease the deformity increases. This lateral deviation, however, does not produce the extensive rotation of the ribs that is seen in true rotary lateral curvature of the spine, due to muscular weakness, faulty positions, and the like.

Secondary compensatory antero-posterior curvatures follow the primary one:

(*a*) In cervical caries we find dorsal incurvation and lumbar excurvation, *a reversal* of the normal physiological curves, and an abnormal flattening of the whole spine in cases of moderate severity. Abnormally short necks are found in severe cases.

(*b*) In dorsal caries we have incurvation above and below the deformity or an *exaggeration* of the normal kyphosis there and the physiological curves.

(*c*) In lumbar disease, we have incurvation above the gibbosity, lessened dorsal kyphosis with a tendency to dorso-lumbar lordosis. Short neck and short trunk are characteristic of severe cervical and dorso-lumbar disease, respectively, when much tissue from the vertebral bodies has been destroyed. We usually find restricted growth of the whole body, but the limbs and head in bad cases seem abnormally long and large, respectively, and the characteristic pinched pained expression of the face in dorsal caries is seen. (Fig. 29.)

We may have arrest of the disease with little or no deformity in the cervical region. Pain and chafing under a brace in the dorsal region may precede increasing deformity or renewed activity of the disease.

The chest is usually thrust forward and downward by dorsal disease and compressed laterally giving rise to "pigeon breast," which may be the first symptom noted as the back is often overlooked. This is explained as an antero-posterior compensatory increase for the loss in the capacity of the chest from above downward. The ribs may be prominent (i. e., protrude beyond) on either side of the sternum and vertebræ, from bending. (Fig. 26.)

6. Grunting Respiration.

This symptom is almost pathognomonic of acute dorsal Pott's Disease. If low down, we will find more thoracic breathing; if high up, more abdominal. Nature thus tries to prevent the ribs jarring the diseased focus and the muscular spasm holds the ribs articulating with the diseased area as motionless as possible.

7. Paralysis.

Paralysis is rarely an early symptom, but may exist without deformity, although this is an exception. (a) Motor paralysis is the rule and varies from a slight fatigue or dragging of the feet at the onset, to an inability to hold one self erect or move the lower extremities at all. About

5.6 per cent of all cases of Pott's Disease have paralysis.   (b)
Sensory paralysis is an indication of very extensive disease
(postero-lateral tracts) as was explained under pathology,
and is rarely if ever complete.   (c) The reflexes, viz: the
knee jerk and ankle clonus, even before the paralysis is

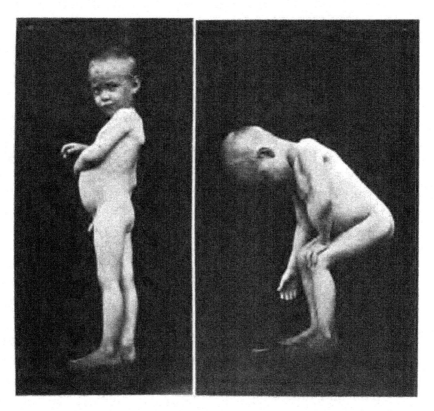

FIG. 31.   FIG. 32.
FIG. 31. LUMBAR DISEASE.
FIG. 32. CHARACTERISTIC METHOD OF STOOPING IN POTT'S DISEASE.

evident, are exaggerated except when the disease is at
the lumbar enlargement; exaggerated reflexes may persist
for some time after locomotion is possible; muscular spasms
may be spontaneous. The muscles become flabby and

powerless, and (*d*) rigidity follows only secondary degenerations. (*e*) Paralysis of the sphincters of the rectum and bladder is present towards the end of all bad cases and those of long duration, and involvement of the lumbar enlargement. (*f*) The arms are paralyzed in a very few cases from extension of the pressure myelitis or pachymeningitis and not usually from ascending secondary degeneration of the cord. (*g*) Trophic and electrical changes in the muscles are rare except when the cervical or lumbar enlargements are involved, then we get atrophy greater than that of disuse and the reaction of degeneration. In severe cases, after prolonged suppuration, we may have a condition of asthenia, with psoas contraction, which may cause a patient to be bedridden without true paralysis. The paralysis is more commonly bilateral and is seen more frequently accompanying *cervical* and *upper dorsal disease*, than the other forms. It rarely lasts more than three years and is usually less than one year in duration if properly treated. The average duration is seven months under efficient treatment. Paralysis is rare (5.6 per cent) under effective treatment, but if present yields readily to it. Extreme pain may precede paralysis. Recurrence of paralysis is rare, though as many as three relapses have been reported. Extreme hyperæsthesia is sometimes present with the sensory paralysis, so that even the bedclothing or hand passed over the paretic region will cause intense pain and muscle spasm.

8. *Abscess.*

Secondary abscess may be cervical, dorsal, mediastinal, axillary, lumbar, iliac, psoas, etc., depending on the seat of the original disease. Psoas abscess, however, is the most frequently seen, even in dorsal disease, as the pus burrows down the sheath of the psoas muscle in the ligamentum arcuatum. Why abscesses should appear externally in some cases and not in others, is not clearly understood, but in some cases (*a*) trauma, such as a fall, blow, etc., may be considered responsible for rekindling the process into activity and increasing its severity, (*b*) lowered vitality may be responsible for abscess in some cases,

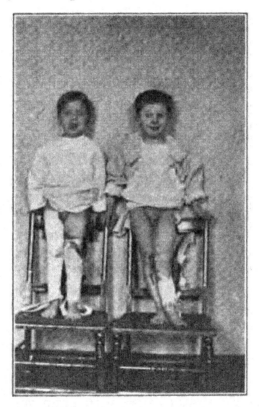

FIG. 33. THE RIGHT HAND CHILD HAS A LEFT TUBERCULAR HIP DISEASE WITH ABSCESS. THE LEFT HAND CHILD HAS POTT'S DISEASE WITH LEFT PSOAS ABSCESS.

as the organism is unable to resist the inroads of the disease; (*c*) imperfect support is responsible in many cases; (*d*) extremely active disease and great numbers of bacilli in others; (*e*) in lumbar disease where secondary abscess is most frequent is explained by the fact that the entire weight of the upper portion of the body is pressing on the diseased focus. (Fig. 33.)

Secondary abscess consists of caseous or calcified masses, necrotic bone trabeculæ in sero-purulent fluid and a few scattered bacilli tuberculosis. It is entirely unlike an acute abscess and is painless except at the time when the primary abscess breaks through the bony wall at its origin, and is known in contradistinction to an acute abscess, as a "cold" abscess. If an abscess bursts into the lung or pleural cavity, it may set up a tuberculous pneumonia, lung abscess or empyema. If into a bronchial tube, it may be coughed up unless extremely large, when it may lead to collapse or apnœa; if into the peritoneum it may cause a tuberculous peritonitis, and into a blood vessel it may result fatally. If it should burst into the hip joint it may start up tuberculous disease there secondarily. It may burrow through into the femoral or inguinal canals and simulate herniæ; these are rare of course. In a very small percentage of cases of cervical or occipito-atloid disease, we may see post-pharyngeal abscess, which need not be considered fatal, as was thought formerly, for this with proper care can be aspirated or it may dribble away, drop by drop, from a small opening and not with a gush, or it may break or be incised on the side of the neck and not lead to strangulation. The lower down in the vertebral column a spinal caries occurs, the more liable is it to be complicated with abscess. As a rule an unopened abscess causes little or no general disturbance and is best left alone unless it reaches such a size as to cause interference with some of the important bodily functions, as perfect drainage and erasion is necessarily impossible. Our main reliance should be in perfect support rather than hasty incision, where perfect drainage is impossible. In certain instances it would seem where the skin is unbroken but thin over a cold abscess, that a hectic condition and *secondary infection* with cocci has occurred. Blood examination gives a *high leucocytosis only* in secondarily

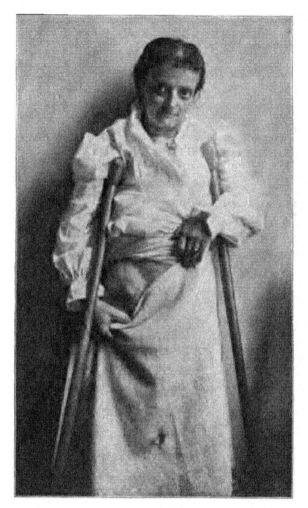

FIG. 34. POTT'S DISEASE WITH ABSCESS COMPLICATING FEMORAL HERNIA.[19]

infected tuberculous abscesses. Secondary infection may occur so readily in an open tuberculous abscess or sinus and

[19] Taylor and Iglehart: Trans., Amer. Orthopædic Assoc., vol. xi, 1898, p. 292.

so often is the cause of the fatal termination of these cases, it cannot be too zealously guarded against. The aureus, albus, streptococcus or colon bacilli will usually be found as the complicating organism.

9. *General Condition.*

The general condition of a patient is more affected from

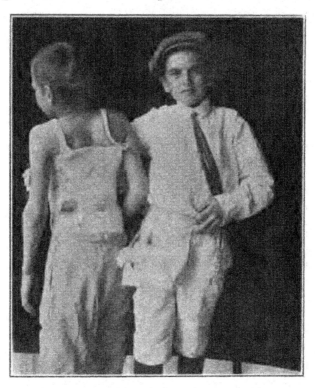

FIG. 35. SINUSES FROM POTT'S DISEASE.

severe Pott's Disease than from any other bone disease. If extensive, it causes retarded growth, often the head and limbs may seem abnormally large and long, respectively, as their growth is not affected by the diseased process as the spine is. The sternum may be very prominent in cases where the deformity is large from collapse of the chest from above down. In some cases, the ribs and cartilages on either side of the sternum may be more prominent than normal and cause the sternum to appear depressed. (Fig. 29.)

Children with this trouble are usually fretful, spoiled and capricious; they are often precocious, but delicate and liable to cold, slight pneumonia, heart trouble and attacks of supposed stomachache, the spinal pain being referred to the peripheral distribution of the sensory nerves.

Tubercular meningitis and general miliary tuberculosis is rarer in this disease than in hip disease. There is in the onset of the disease, little or no general disturbance, but as the disease advances, we will find the appetite, nutrition, sleep and other normal functions of the body seriously impaired.

In those cases which have sinuses (often secondarily infected) discharging for a long period of time, months or even years, a cachexia ensues, the patient has a waxy color, amyloid changes may occur in the viscera, œdema and dropsy ensue, and a secondary anæmia be noted in the red and white blood cells. (Fig. 36.)

10. *Temperature.*

In all cases where the disease has established a footing, there is more or less elevation of temperature. This rarely if ever amounts to a hyper-pyrexia, and we may say as a rule that the temperature of tubercular bone disease varies from a subnormal morning temperature to $99\frac{1}{2}°$ to 101° F. in the afternoon. When however a secondary abscess occurs with a discharging sinus and this sinus and abscess cavity become secondarily infected with pyogenic bacteria, "hectic fever" sets in, with a low morning temperature and high evening temperature (102° to 105° F.) with chilly sensations, sweats and the characteristic "hectic flush" in the cheeks.

DIAGNOSIS.

The diagnosis is made by considering the symptoms mentioned, such as: (1) Stiffness of the neck or back with marked muscular spasm; peculiar attitude and gait; (2) night cries; (3) seat and localization of the pain and the character

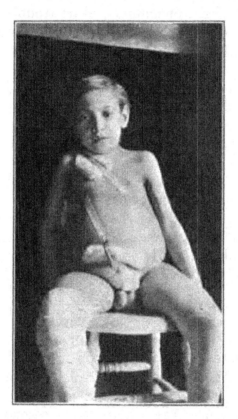

FIG. 36. AMYLOID DISEASE OF THE VISCERA COMPLICATING MULTIPLE TUBER-
CULAR BONE LESIONS WITH SECONDARY INFECTIONS. DROPSY.

of the nervous symptoms; (4) prominence and irregularity in the line of the spinous processes; (5) psoas contraction in dorso-lumbar disease and grunting respiration in acute dorsal disease; (6) abscess; (7) temperature; together with

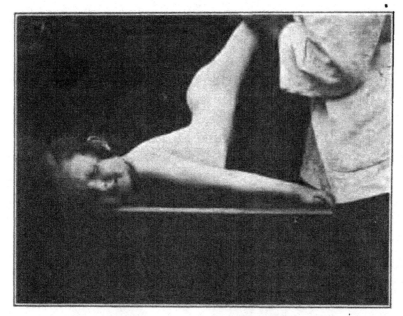

FIG. 37 A NORMAL FLEXIBLE SPINE.

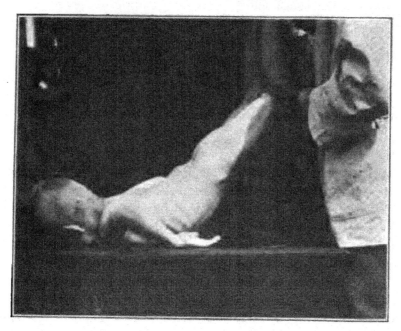

FIG. 38. A RIGID SPINE IN POTT'S DISEASE.

(8) family history; (9) the skiagraph; (10) the blood count; (11) the insidious onset; (12) the tuberculin test.

Stiffness of the spinal muscles is easily made manifest by requesting the child to stoop and pick anything up, which it will do without bending the back; (Fig. 32) the same may be said of its efforts to touch its toes when sitting. When lying on its face, if the examiner attempts to raise the child from the examining table by its feet, instead of the back arching anteriorly as it does normally into a perfect

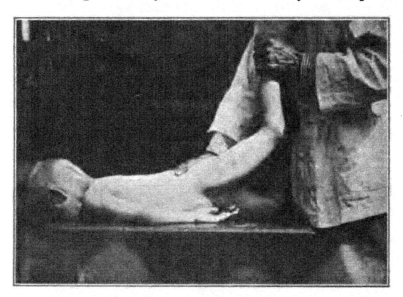

FIG. 39. A TEST FOR PSOAS CONTRACTION.

bow, it will be held flat. (Figs. 37 and 38.) There is also no lateral flexibility. We can demonstrate the spasm of the erector spinæ group by raising the child when his hands and feet are touching the floor, by placing one's hands under the abdomen when the spine will be held flat and rigid (Whitman's sign). Psoas contraction is easily diagnosticated by having the child lie on its face and flexing its legs at a right angle with its thighs, so that resistance will be detected in one leg when the examiner extends first one leg and then the other, by raising them alternately from the examining table, when the hand is held over the sacrum. (Fig. 39.) Psoas spasm can also be shown by allowing the child to

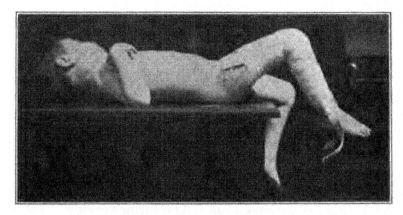

FIG. 40. WHITMAN'S TEST FOR PSOAS CONTRACTION.

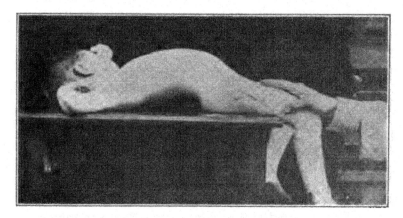

FIG. 41. WHITMAN'S TEST FOR PSOAS CONTRACTION.
(Note arched Lumbar Spine as the flexed leg from the contracted Psoas Muscle is pulled down to the table.)

sit on the edge of a table and let the legs hang down, the normal leg will hang lower than the affected one (Whitman). Of course if both legs are rigidly flexed on the abdomen one cannot get such a patient to lie flat on the abdomen in making the usual test. (Fig. 39.) Psoas spasm is a valuable sign in commencing lower dorsal and lumbar disease, as well as beginning abscess and becomes more pronounced as the disease becomes more extensive. The iliac fossæ should be carefully palpated and percussed for abscess as a matter of routine in all cases of lower dorsal and lumbar Pott's Disease and percussion and auscultation should be employed over the posterior mediastinum in suspected abscess of the dorsal region. Careful palpation in beginning curves of the most prominent spinous process may show that it is more movable than the adjacent ones, owing to the softening and disintegration of the intervertebral ligaments and may elicit pain. (Whitman.) In doubtful cases a blood count and X-ray photograph are to be used to help clear up the diagnosis. The former giving negative information as the red cells show a secondary anæmia in advanced disease only and leucocytosis of the white elements only in secondary infection of tuberculous abscess cavities by the pyogenic bacteria. The X-ray, on the other hand, shows *a clouding of the tuberculous area, loss of the quadrilateral shape of the vertebral bodies* and *absence of the clear spaces, which indicate the intervertebral cartilages.* (Fig. 42.) The tuberculin test can be used *only* in conjunction with *several of the clinical symptoms* above mentioned, for otherwise a positive reaction, viz: an elevation of 2° over the usual temperature and chilliness, nausea, headache or muscular pains would not locate the tubercular disease; too small a dose will not give the reaction; other diseases may give a positive reaction, and the author considers it of less value as a means of diagnosis in this manifestation of tuberculosis than the others named. There may or may not be increase in the acuteness of symptoms referable to the point of disease.

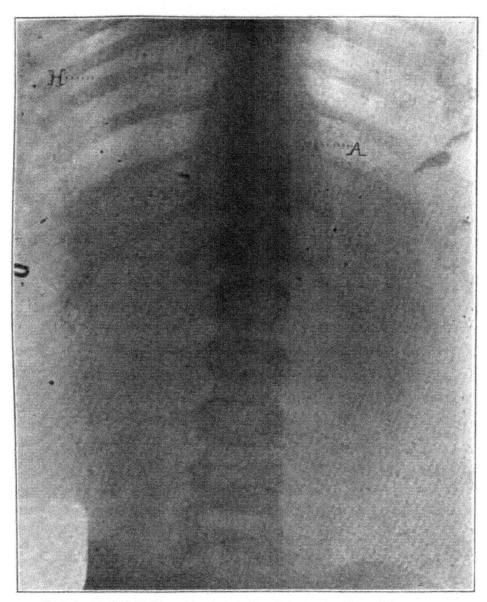

FIG. 42. CASE OF TUBERCULOSIS OF THE SPINE, SHOWING LOSS OF THE NORMAL OUTLINE OF THE BODIES AND DISCS, AT THE TENTH AND ELEVENTH DORSAL VERTEBRÆ. ABSCESS SHADOW (A) AS WELL AS HEART SHADOW (H) IS SHOWN.

DIFFERENTIAL DIAGNOSIS.

1. *Torticollis:* In simple chronic torticollis, the contraction is more commonly of the sterno-cleido-mastoid and trapezius muscles, predominating at any rate and no pain is present. In caries all the muscles are contracted, especially the posterior cervicals and deep groups. The patient also in beginning and acute caries of the cervical vertebræ supports and protects the head from jar and cannot move it in either direction without pain.

2. Functional Neuroses, Railroad Spine, Typhoid Spine, etc., are rare in children. In these conditions we find tender points over the spines and usually get a history of traumatism or previous disease. In caries this tenderness over the spine is not the rule and the characteristic deformity and muscle spasm are present even at an early stage.

4. From Trauma, Rheumatism, and Strain in children the diagnosis of Pott's Disease is to be made with caution. The former tend to spontaneous recovery, while caries untreated gets worse. In adults caries is rare as compared with its frequency in children. It is to be borne in mind, however, that the pain and other symptoms of tuberculous spondylitis quiet down also with treatment, so that suspicious cases should not too soon be considered simple sprains and ample means of diagnosis should be availed of. One sees occasionally rupture of the posterior spinous ligaments and the diagnosis of this ¡condition can be made by the greater separation of the spinous processes at a point of tenderness after injury. (Painter.) True rheumatism has a family history of that disease, the temperature is higher than in Pott's Disease, the onset is sudden and other joints are involved.

4. Rickets shows a longer curve in the dorso-lumbar region. It may be sharp and angular, however, with some spinal stiffness, but the other signs of rickets are present,

and the children are very young.   Pain and night cries are absent.

5. Lateral Curvature following tubercular osteitis does not show so much rotation of the ribs as in the simple form due to muscular atony.   It is usually a late symptom; but may be early and associated with the other symptoms of Pott's Disease, however.   In early cases, several careful examinations may be necessary to establish a diagnosis, between the muscular or tuberculous forms of slight scoliosis.

6. Tubercular hip disease gives a limitation of flexion, adduction, abduction and rotation as well as of extension of the thigh, which last is the only motion of the hip joint limited in dorso-lumbar caries with the exception of possibly rotation.

7. Carcinoma of the spine rarely occurs in children and in adults is a secondary manifestation of cancer elsewhere. It may have all the symptoms of tuberculous spinal disease, but is so very unusually seen that other signs of malignant disease elsewhere in the body would attract one's attention first.

8. Primary sarcoma in children is one of the rarest of diseases and may be eliminated from ordinary consideration.

9. Meningeal tumors cause paralysis of various forms, but do not affect the vertebral bodies, except late in this disease by absorption, only then causing changes in attitude and carriage.   The diagnosis is to be made by the clinical history.

10. Aneurism with absorption of portions of the vertebral bodies is to be diagnosticated by auscultation, which means of diagnosis should be availed of in orthopædic practice as a routine, as well as inspection, palpation, percussion, etc.

11. Primary gummata of spinal vertebræ are not recorded, as the more usual osseous specific lesion is periosteal or at the junction of epiphysis and diaphysis in the long bones,

associated with enlarged spleen and glands and secondary anæmia.

12. Rheumatoid arthritis may have stiffness of the spine and pain in the area of exostoses and peripheral nerve distribution, with a less degree of muscular spasm and no characteristic projection of the spinous processes. The cervical spine is most usually attacked in this disease, but the ribs may be ankylosed to the spine in the dorsal form, so that the chest cannot expand well, or the whole spine may be involved. It is more commonly a disease of advanced life, chiefly in women, than of childhood.

13. Perinephritis, appendicitis, sacro-iliac disease and caries of the sacrum show only one or two of the symptoms of spinal caries and should never be mistaken for it.

14. Acute processes are diagnosticated from Pott's Disease by high leucocytosis, sudden onset and the high temperatures present.

PROGNOSIS.

The prognosis for spontaneous recovery in untreated cases is good, though tedious and the symptoms may be severe and deformity extreme. With efficient treatment the prognosis is very favorable. The mortality is greater in adults than in children, but the statistics as to death from this disease are imperfect, and is given at about 25 per cent of all cases and perhaps 5 per cent in the treated cases. The average duration of life is about fifty years.

Causes of Death. (1) Asthenia from lowered vitality in prolonged disease, torsion or stenosis of the aorta and heart disease; (2) paralysis, rarely; (3) phthisis; (4) amyloid disease of viscera, and (5) fatty degeneration of viscera from prolonged suppuration of secondarily infected abscesses and sinuses; (6) general miliary tuberculosis or tuberculous meningitis; (7) bursting of an abscess into the larynx, lungs, posterior mediastinum, pleura, peritoneum, œsophagus, spinal canal or into a blood vessel; (8) serious intercurrent disease, such as scarlet fever, on a system already devitalized, have all been reported as causes of death.

PROGNOSIS AS TO ABSCESS.

The chances are 50 to 1 in lumbar disease that secondary abscess will appear, 25 to 1 in dorsal disease and 1 to 50 in cervical disease. From 12 to 25 per cent of all cases have abscess. Abscess in adults is more unfavorable than in children, but depends on the site, drainage or completeness of evacuation, or upon the vitality of the individual, when unopened. Abscess usually indicates severe cases. Psoas abscess with contraction adds to the difficulty of and length of time for treatment. Many abscesses are of such small size that they escape detection in life, as they cause no symptoms. All cases may be said to have abscess, but when the term is used, it refers to one of appreciable size or the secondary abscess outside of the original bone focus.

Phthisis pulmonalis is more common in adults. Recession of the deformity is apparent in some cases from ankylosis of the diseased vertebræ and the greater growth of the healthy adjacent ones; the kyphosis is then proportionately less prominent. As a rule, however, the kyphosis increases during the growing years as do the compensatory curves.

PROGNOSIS AS TO DURATION.

The time required for treatment depends on: (1) the general health of the patient; (2) the size, the region and the amount of the spine diseased; and (3) the amount of the superincumbent weight; as a rule not less than three years. The cervical naturally takes less long to heal than lumbar disease. Protection for firm ankylosis requires a long time, especially is this true in growing children. At puberty there seems to be a danger of redevelopment of the symptoms, therefore care and protection of the spine is especially necessary then.

PROGNOSIS IN PARALYSIS.

Prognosis as to the time of recovery from paralysis, under efficient treatment, is from seven months to one year. Recovery may occur suddenly, from the evacuation of an abscess, hyperextension of the spine, forcible reduction of the deformity with relief of the stenosis of spinal vessels from œdematous pressure, etc.

The prognosis, if sensation is abolished, especially if there is paralysis of the rectum and bladder, is less favorable and very much less favorable in amyloid disease.

THE PRINCIPLES OF TREATMENT.

The principles of treatment are rest and immobilization, which are accomplished by (1) recumbency, (2) traction, and (3) fixation, *with the spine hyperextended* at the point of disease. These principles of treatment are based on the following facts: First, if we review briefly some of the chief anatomical features of the spine we find the vertebral column as a whole consists of four curves when viewed laterally—a convexity forward in the cervical region, a convexity backward in the dorsal region, a convexity again forward in the lumbar region and backward in the sacral.

The three first-mentioned curves, with which only we are concerned, are subject to variations dependent on whether the individual is standing or sitting, and also whether the observation is made on rising in the morning or late in the evening, being in the latter cases more marked.

It has been shown by Brackett[20] that recumbency in a prone position lessens these curves, and supine recumbency has been used from time immemorial as an efficient means of treating spinal curvatures.

[20] Bradford and Lovett: Orthopædic Surgery, 2d ed., 1899, 53.

Suspension by the head and hands also straightens out these physiological curves, if we may so designate them. Le Vacher[21] first demonstrated this in 1768, in his "L'arbor suspendens" attached to a corset.

Very similar to Le Vacher's "L'arbor suspendens," is the "jury mast," for which Lee gives the credit to J. K. Mitchell in 1826, and Lee's own "self-suspension spinal swing," devised in 1866, confirmed this observation in regard to the physiological curves. The elder Sayre is often credited with the jury mast, however, and also the spinal swing. We know now that these physiological curves are chiefly lessened by suspension and not the curves due to tubercular disease, as earlier observers thought.

In the erect posture, the spine must bear the superincumbent weight of the head and by means of the ribs and diaphragm also the weight of the thoracic viscera, and, to a certain extent, the liver and other abdominal organs. Further, through the sternal attachments of the shoulder girdle and the anterior situation of the arms, there is to a certain extent also a drag downward and forward on the dorsal spine by them.

If the spine, as a whole, is viewed in profile in either a skeleton or a fresh specimen, it will be seen that a vertical line drawn through the bodies of the cervical vertebræ will pass anterior to the dorsal vertebræ, not touching them, but in the lumbar region such a line will again reach the vertebral bodies. Thus, from an anatomical standpoint, we may conclude that the mechanics of the spinal column decidedly predispose to a dorsal convexity, or kyphosis, even without the addition of disease, which the continuity of the vertebral bodies and intervertebral fibrocartilages antagonize anteriorly and the ligamenta flava, inter and supraspinalia and muscles posteriorly.

[21] Memoirs de l'Académie royale de Chirurgie, Paris, 1768, tome 4.

Secondly. From the pathological findings in caries of
the vertebræ since the time of Sir Percival Pott, observers
have noted that the less compact bodies of the vertebræ
are the seat of the tubercular osteitis, softening and disintegration and not the denser articular and transverse processes, as a rule. As a result of this in untreated, mal-
treated and neglected cases, the characteristic deformity
has occurred, i. e., the superior and inferior edges of the
bodies of the involved vertebræ have come into closer
contact anteriorly and the spinous processes are more widely
separated than is normal. In addition, unless means are
adopted to check this, the healthy vertebral bodies will
come into contact with those diseased and from the traumatic irritation produced thereby and the contiguity, the
healthy vertebræ will also become involved in the process
and so the diseased area will extend.

What, then, can we gather from this, as the indication
for treatment to combat this normal and pathological tendency to kyphosis? (Fig. 43.)

Manifestly it is the maintenance of hyperextension of
the spine until all danger of extension of the tubercular
process is passed and firm cicatrization has occurred with
a layer of non-tubercular granulation tissue, which is
converted in time into fibrous tissue, cartilage or bone, or
a formative osteitis locks the vertebral bodies or processes
together inseparably by ankylosis.

I have illustrated this diagrammatically: Let Fig. 43 A
represent two healthy vertebræ seen in profile. The parallel lines represent the superior and inferior planes of those
bodies. The center of gravity or weight-bearing line is
indicated by the dotted line, seen to pass through the center
of the vertebral bodies. The alignment of the spinous processes is seen to be straight.

In Fig. 43 B we see the result of an untreated tubercular

process where the bodies have collapsed, the planes of the superior and inferior surfaces converge and meet anterior to the vertebral column and the spinous processes are widely separated. The center of gravity line is thrown further forward, tending to increase the deformity. The separation of the spinous processes shows the characteristic contour of the humpback.

In Fig. 43c is shown what should be the aim of treatment, viz: the separation of the vertebral bodies as far as the liga-

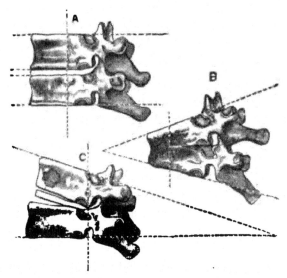

FIG. 43. DIAGRAMMATIC REPRESENTATION OF THE PRODUCTION OF THE DEFORMITY OF POTT'S DISEASE. A, NORMAL. B, POTT'S DISEASE. AND C, AIM OF TREATMENT.

mentous and muscular attachments will permit, the throwing of the center of gravity back on the articular processes and the crowding together of the spinous processes.

We cannot say that a true separation of the vertebral bodies really occurs by hyperextension before extensive bone destruction has taken place, but certainly intervertebral pressure is lessened and in extensive unhealed disease, where softening of the tissues still·exists, such a separation certainly occurs in hyperextension. With these principles before us we are now in a position to take up

TREATMENT IN DETAIL.

Recumbency: The patient is to be placed prone on the face or supine on the back on a *firm* mattress; if on the back, the head is to be low and a pad under the deformity is to be used to separate the diseased vertebral bodies as much as possible by hyperextension of the spine. The patient is not to be allowed to sit up nor lie on the side, as these postures twist and move the spine, nor is the patient to bend forward for such motion crowds the vertebral bodies together producing trauma at the disease softened area. As a means of fixation or to accomplish the methods laid down above, we may use the Bradford bed frame, which accomplishes many of the objects to be found serviceable in recumbency; offers the further advantage of making the patient portable and renders out-of-door life on this stretcher more simple.

Hyperextension may be accomplished by felt or hair cushions or padded wooden blocks, or by bending the Bradford frame upward into an arch, as suggested by Whitman, in order to produce lordosis as much as possible at the seat of disease.

The author prefers the padded wooden blocks under the deformity as enabling one more accurately to localize the hyperextension. A plaster of paris jacket applied in hyperextension is sometimes necessary in addition to the Bradford frame for the recumbent treatment of restless children.

TRACTION.

Traction in recumbency for acute cases is most useful. A padded webbing sling under the chin and occiput attached to a spreader and cord with a weight of one-half to five pounds is used, or a regular Sayre leather head sling may be employed.

Counter extension in cervical cases is afforded by the body weight on raising the head of the bed. In acute lumbar cases, a double Buck's extension to both legs and raising the foot of the bed will be found useful. Recumbency will be found more applicable and better tolerated in children than in adults. Recumbency should be thorough, fixation perfect and no half measures used, as we then get the dangers and disadvantages of confinement without thorough treatment. (Fig. 9.)

Traction is employed to relieve pain or paralysis. In paralysis or severely painful cases traction on the head and legs both should be employed. It has been proven, however, that traction cannot pull the vertebræ apart except where the disease is extensive, but it does diminish intervertebral pressure and overcomes muscular spasm. Whether deformity has occurred or not the small firm pads or pillows should be fastened to the undershirt on either side of the diseased region over the transverse processes, or used separately as a padded block of wood with a groove down its center to avoid excoriating the skin over the spinous processes, in order to exert an upward pressure and antagonize deformity, when the child is recumbent and to maintain hyperextension. Pads of curled hair or the best piano or sadler's felt, are the most useful materials to employ.

The objections to recumbency are: (1) the confinement; (2) the restlessness of the patient; and (3) it seems to produce a tendency to meningitis when too long continued, probably from lowered vitality incident to the confinement.

Recumbency is indicated and necessary in (1) acute cases; (2) paralysis; (3) abscess, when painful or causing contractions; (4) those cases which are easily tired; (5) high cervical cases; (6) low dorsal or lumbar disease; (7) as a routine treatment in all cases in the early period of disease and *for a certain period daily throughout the disease.* Even after a week of recumbency improvement is generally noted in appetite, increased weight, absence of pain and improvement in general condition. Recumbency for a month or six weeks in the early stages of the disease will be found extremely helpful in this disease and should be continued until the acute symptoms subside.

TREATMENT BY SUSPENSION.

Absolute suspension of the body by the neck, *i. e.*, "hanging," by means of a head sling can be used only, temporarily of course. Continuous head suspension or traction or support, as we may call it, can be obtained and is *always necessary* and to be used in *cervical* and *high dorsal* caries to remove the superincumbent weight from the diseased spine, by the jury mast, the various head supports and collars in conjunction with spinal corsets or braces to be described later. This head suspension is a most essential part of treatment in the regions named and without it deformity surely ensues.

FIXATIVE AND SUPPORTING TREATMENT.

This means of treatment is secured by corsets or jackets of plaster of paris, paper, wood, aluminum, leather, celluloid, etc., and the different varieties of steel spinal braces.

There are five methods of applying plaster of paris jackets, (*a*) the Sayre suspension and traction method; (*b*) the Brackett recumbent and extension method; (*c*) pads or support under the chest and pelvis; (*d*) manual suspension, and (*e*) the writer's method of partial suspension and hyperextension with the patient in a sitting attitude, or of hyperextension and traction while recumbent.

PREPARATION OF THE PATIENT FOR A JACKET.

Before describing these methods in detail, it may be well to give a few suggestions on the preparation of the patient.

The child should be stripped of all the clothes and the body bathed with 95 per cent alcohol to harden the skin. A summer weight undershirt or seamless stockinet should then be put on that extends well up in the neck and down below the trochanters. It is to be pinned tightly over the shoulders and under the perineum. If any deformity exists, pads of superimposed layers of piano felt, about an inch and a half wide and of sufficient length to extend all along the bony prominence, should be stitched to the shirt over the transverse processes on either side of the affected region and sufficiently close together to prevent the plaster jacket, when hardened, from rubbing and ulcerating the skin over the prominent spinous processes. If this precaution is not taken, a troublesome sore may result. If the child is very thin, it may be necessary to put piano felt pads over the anterior superior spines of the ilia and sternum to prevent excoriation. When this is done, the child is ready for the application of the jacket, which is done with turns of wet plaster of paris bandages. Formerly a pad, called a "dinner pad," was placed over the abdomen and withdrawn after the jacket hardened, but this is unnecessary.

Now, we will consider methods of applying plaster of paris jackets. There are many different ways of accomplishing this, which the author has found useful, depending on the case.

(a) The Sayre Method.

The oldest or (a) Sayre method makes use of an apparatus consisting of a head sling and straps which pass under the axillæ; these are supported by a spreader, which is attached to a rope with a pulley in the ceiling by means of which the patient can be suspended and any desired degree of traction made and the jacket applied. Formerly, it was considered by some, that it was possible to straighten out the deformity by this suspension; this, however, is not the case; the superin-

cumbent weight is removed and the spine is lengthened
in so far as the physiological curves are straightened out,
but the pathological curves are not. The jacket acts as a
means of fixation of the spinal column and prevents any
bending forward, which would cause additional damage to
the already diseased vertebræ. The bandages are simply
wound smoothly without tension around the body until the
judgment prompts one that a sufficient number have been
used to furnish the necessary thickness to support the
individual case. If by this method, as may be found, the
jacket does not fit tightly over the sternum, "V's" may be
cut out of the top (wide end up) with the plaster knife and
the edges of the "V's" approximated by additional turns of
plaster bandages. A possible objection to this method may
be the nervousness and fright of a child at being suspended
or "hung," as they call it, but it certainly is of value in many
acute cases for the relief of pain, in that it removes the
superincumbent weight. It is also of value in cases where
the deformity is due as much to the exaggeration of the
physiological curves as to the deformity itself. The chief
objection is the unsteadiness and swaying of the patient
during the application of the jacket and that it produces no
hyperextension of the spine.

(b) Davy-Brackett Hammock Method.

This method enables us to put a jacket on a child in recumbency. The apparatus consists of a quadrilateral gas pipe
frame, 6 x 3 feet in dimension, in which, by means of a screw
attached to a rod passing through one end of a flat hammock
composed of twill cotton, the other end being made fast to
the frame, it may be drawn taut; on this the patient is
allowed to lie on his face. Slits are made on either side of
the patient's body in the twill cotton, usually the portion
of the hammock remaining under the patient's body, being

sufficiently strong to maintain the weight; it is then a matter of no difficulty winding the plaster bandages around the hammock and patient until the jacket is completed. Difficulty arises in this method from the upper part of the sternum not touching the hammock, so that it is impossible on a tight hammock to have the jacket fit snugly against *the upper part of the thorax*, where it is *so essential to prevent flexion of the spine forward* in its upper dorsal segment, which

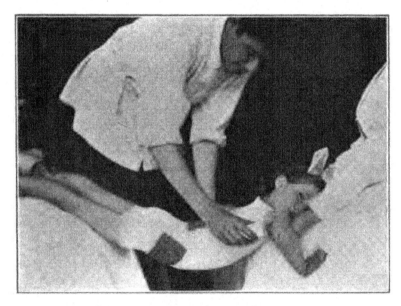

FIG. 44. MANUAL METHOD OF APPLYING JACKET.

would manifestly defeat the aim of treatment; this can be obviated in the same way as that suggested in jackets applied by the Sayre method of cutting out "V's" at the top; or the lower part of a jacket may be applied, the hammock cut through at the top and the child held by the arms or shoulders, while the upper part of the jacket is completed, and then the hammock at the lower part can be cut through. This, however, is apt to leave an uncomfortable ridge in the middle.   Or a hole can be cut for the face to go through and thus bring the sternum in contact with the hammock.   It is an easy matter to pull out the piece of hammock from within the jacket, almost always, after it is cut across at the top and bottom.   (Fig. 45.)

(c) Chest-pelvic Support Method.

Two boxes or sandbags or supports of any kind may be used one under the child's sternum when lying face down and one under the thighs and the bandages can then be

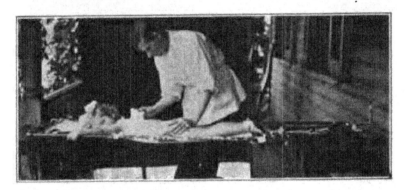

FIG. 45   BRACKETT HAMMOCK.

applied.   Manifestly a jacket applied in this crude way should be finished later at the top, when the child can stand, in order to come up high on the sternum.

(d) Manual Suspension.

A very simple, efficient and ready way, when no other means are at hand, is to have one assistant grasp the child's arms when lying face down, and a second assistant grasp the thighs and swing the child horizontally between them, when the surgeon can apply the jacket.   Hyperextension and a very snug jacket can thus be obtained.   (Fig. 44.)

(e) *The Method of Hyperextension.*

To meet the aims of treatment, previously outlined, in the latter part of 1894, the author presented before the Johns Hopkins Medical Society[22] what he termed an apparatus for applying plaster jackets on a plaster jacket stool surmounted by a bicycle saddle, on which the patient sat, with the pelvis fixed, the arms extended upward and backward to hand grips dependent from a vertical posterior upright and traction was made on the head by means of a head sling attached to cord and pulley on the posterior upright. The feet were supported on rigid adjustable stirrups. The result of this attitude on the spine was lordosis. In that paper, as far as one can find out in the literature, attention was first called to and the importance demonstrated clinically of extending the spine backward (hyperextension) and the maintenance of this position by means of plaster of paris jackets for the prevention or correction of the natural tendency of the deformity of Pott's Disease. Hadra, in 1891, suggested for fracture but not Pott's Disease the same principle by wiring the spinous processes together, "thereby relieving the vertebral bodies."[23] Other methods to accomplish the same end were published by other observers shortly after.

Chipault published on March 9, 1895, his method of wiring the spinous and transverse processes in Pott's Disease after "forcible correction" of the deformity under anæsthesia, which consisted in manual traction by several surgeons and assistants on the head and extremities and pressure on the gibbosity, preparatory to applying plaster of paris.

Calot published a paper on similar operations in 1896[24] and his name and not Chipault's is associated with the operation of "forcible correction."

[22] Johns Hopkins Bulletin, No. 45, February, 1895, and Medical News, March 23, 1895.
[23] Hadra: Trans. Amer. Ortho. Assoc., vol. iv, 205.
[24] Calot: Trans. Acad. Med., Paris, 1896.

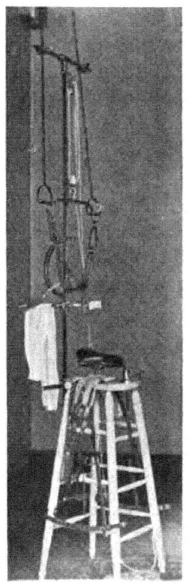

FIG. 46.   UPRIGHT KYPHOTONE·

Goldthwait reported, in 1898, his and Metzger's excellent method of hyperextension, without anæsthesia, in which the patient lies supine on two strips of steel, that portion of the spine above the knuckle being unsupported and gravity acting as the correcting force.[25]   The jacket is then applied.

Redard in the same year published his method of mechanical traction in a prone position with anæsthesia and manual pressure on the boss.[26]

In 1898 the author presented to the American Orthopædic Association[27] his plaster jacket stool of 1894, supplemented with a pressure rod, to control the point at which hyperextension was to be made (viz: at the kyphosis) and called the apparatus the kyphotone (κύφος, hunchback, and τεινεῖν, to extend).   It had been found that without pressure on the knuckle in mid-dorsal cases, the lordosis, or hyperextension, frequently was more marked in the lumbar region

[25] Goldthwait: Trans. Amer. Ortho. Assoc., vol. ix, 1899; Boston Med. and Surg. Jour., July 28, 1898.
[26] Redard: Archivo di Orthopedia, 1898, Fasc. 2.
[27] Transactions, vol. xii, and N. Y. Med. Jour., May 12, 1900, 716.

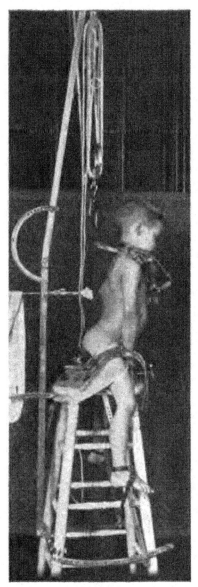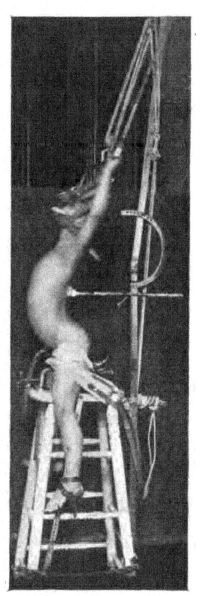

FIG. 47.   FIG. 48.

FIG 47. UPRIGHT KYPHOTONE, SHOWING A CASE OF POTT'S DISEASE.
FIG. 48. SAME CASE WITH KYPHOTONE IN ACTION.

than in the region of disease ànd more marked than was desirable, but the pressure rod on the knuckle obviated this,

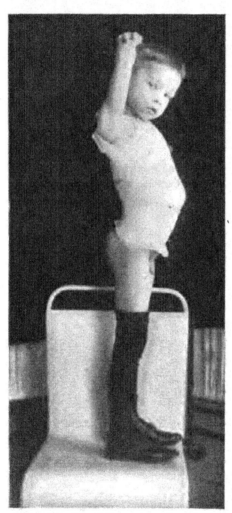

FIG. 49. SAME CASE WITH RESULTING JACKET AND CORRECTION OF DEFORMITY. "SUMMER" OR "FIGURE OF 8" JACKET.

making *the region of the gibbosity* the center of this arc. (Figs. 46, 47, 48 and 49.)

The comparative value of suspension and hyperextension in the correction of the deformity of Pott's Disease is well shown in photographs. In a double photographic exposure the lower photograph shows the child sitting on the kyphotone and the large knuckle is well seen against the background. The upper photograph shows the child suspended by the Sayre head sling only and the knuckle is virtually of the same size it was before traction was made. In another picture of the same child, taken at the same time, we see traction has been made on

the head, the arms have been carried upwards and backwards, the pelvis has been made fast by the wide webbing strap and the pressure rod has been applied, causing hyper-extension at the knuckle, with the result that the spine is virtually straight. (Figs. 50 and 51.) In Fig. 52 we see this patient cured with a straight spine.

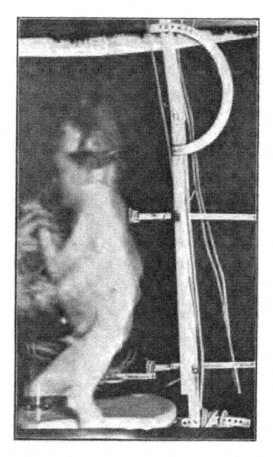

FIG. 50. DOUBLE PHOTOGRAPHIC EXPOSURE OF A CASE OF POTT'S DISEASE WITH-OUT AND WITH TRACTION ON THE SPINE BUT NO HYPEREXTENSION. THE DEFORMITY IS UNCHANGED.

The author presented also two recumbent kyphotones at the same time, which carry out the same mechanical principles of hyperextension.

The larger is similar in many details to the one attached
to the office stool, but differs in having the patient lie in a
supine position on a plate or pelvic crutch instead of sitting
up.   The main bar slides in a solid metal block and thus

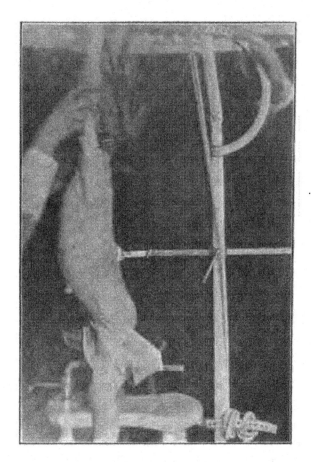

FIG. 51.   SAME CASE AS SHOWN IN FIG. 50, SHOWING RESULT OF HYPEREXTENSION
MADE AT SAME SITTING.

can be lengthened or shortened to adapt itself to the patient's
size.   The pressure rod, attachments for hands and head
sling are similar to the upright kyphotone.   (Fig. 53.)

The smaller kyphotone is quite simple, inexpensive and can be easily taken apart and carried in a satchel to a patient's house. It consists of two solid bases and uprights, one surmounted by a plate of sufficient size to support the pelvis and the second by a small plate to press upwards against the knuckle, when the patient lies supine. The small plate is adjustable and can be raised or lowered to increase the pressure on the kyphos and vice versa. The distance between the uprights can also be regulated by a rod attached to the bases by setscrews. (Figs. 54 and 55.) The plate of the pressure rod is incorporated in the plaster jacket during its application but can be easily slipped out after the patient is removed from the machine by making an incision on one side of the pressure rod in the plaster, which at this stage has not entirely hardened. Then the opening thus made can be entirely and easily closed by molding together the moist edges. Or preferably the patient is pulled upward or forward depending on which kyphotone is used, as the bandage is rolled between the plate and the spine (McKim's modification).

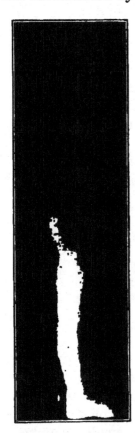

FIG. 52. SAME BOY AS SHOWN IN FIG. 50 AS HE IS TODAY. CURED WITHOUT DEFORMITY.

Both of these recumbent kyphotones were made to meet the need of acute or early cases or those with external pachymeningitis with paraplegic symptoms, in which it is detrimental to even sit up momentarily, until the head sling is adjusted and the superincumbent weight removed.

The question of which of these machines we shall use to prevent, correct or improve the deformity of Pott's Disease depends on the pathological condition we find in the spine, as shown by its flexibility, the size of the knuckle not necessarily being a determining factor of the latter; in other words, *prior to ankylosis, the spine can be made much straighter,* by hyperextension at the point of the kyphosis.

(1) *Earliest Stages.* At this period there is little or no deformity to correct, but the child will indicate by its pos-

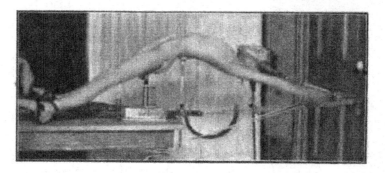

FIG. 53. LARGE RECUMBENT KYPHOTONE IN ACTION.

ture, carriage or gait, grunting respiration, pain, night cries, muscular spasm or some of the characteristic symptoms, that spinal trouble is present. The region can be located and prevention of deformity obtained by plaster jackets applied in slight hyperextension on the small recumbent kyphotone.

At this stage caseation and conglomeration of the tubercles is beginning and traumatic contact from pressure of the healthy adjacent vertebræ is ripe to help break down the diseased vertebral body.

(2) *Beginning Deformity.* In such a case the vertebral body has partially broken down and abscess formation has

begun. Correction may be obtained by gravity with the small or large recumbent kyphotone or upright kyphotone and maintained by a plaster jacket.

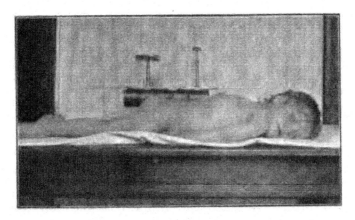

Fig. 54. Small Recumbent Kyphotone.

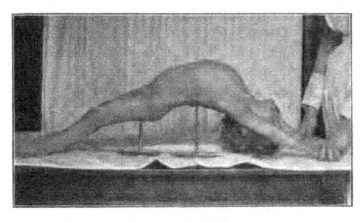

Fig. 55. Small Recumbent Kyphotone in Action.
Same Child as Shown in Fig. 54.

(3) *More Advanced Cases.* In a case in which several vertebral bodies have broken down, and in which some adhesions or fibrous ankylosis are just starting to form, either the large recumbent or preferably the upright kypho-

tone may be necessary to correct, with head sling traction and pelvic fixation. It is at times astonishing to see a large hump disappear under this treatment, perhaps not at one sitting but by degrees, as a series of jackets are applied month after month.

(4) *Neglected or Ankylosed Cases.* If the ankylosis in a case is solid and condensing osteitis has taken place, no extreme force is justifiable. Pain should be the guide to the amount of pressure or traction force used. Even, however, in large knuckles or humps, it may be found the ankylosis is not so solid as one would be led to think and it is certainly justifiable to lessen the deformity of such a case by one of the more powerful kyphotones and allow the spine to heal in an improved position.

In low lumbar disease the hammock method may be preferable or the recumbent kyphotones with a spica on each thigh.

The method suggested by Bradford and Vose[28] would seem also applicable to the first two of the foregoing varieties. This method consists of allowing the child to lie on its back and be slung in a position of hyperextension by a piece of firm cloth passing under the kyphos. This cloth, after passing around the sides and back is attached to a pulley, by means of which the hyperextension of the spine can be regulated.

AN EFFICIENT AND INEXPENSIVE KYPHOTONE.

My original kyphotone was rather expensive and complicated, so that in the summer of 1905 I had made for our Mountain Hospital for Surgical Tuberculosis, by a blacksmith, the one herewith presented for seven dollars and a half, which answers every purpose and which anyone could duplicate anywhere. (Fig. 56.)

[28] Annals of Surgery, 1899, vol. xvii, 223.

It has a gas pipe base supporting a wooden seat and pelvic clamp with a steel upright holding a horseshoe-shaped hand grip and a pressure rod.

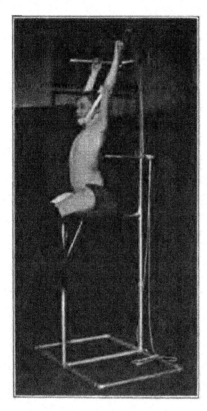

FIG. 56. INEXPENSIVE UPRIGHT KYPHOTONE.

Each of the last two named are easily adjustable for each case by simply turning one thumbscrew on each.

The gas pipe base is three feet wide, two feet deep and three feet high; the posterior upright is four feet long, making the entire apparatus seven feet high. The horseshoe-shaped hand grip is thirty-six inches long and the pressure rod is eighteen inches long.

The seat is eighteen inches wide by twelve inches deep, fastened by bolts to the gas pipe and can be moved forwards or backwards, depending on the size of the patient. In the center of the seat (not shown in the cut) is a buffer of wood, 2 x 4 x 3 inches, which is a point of counter pressure against the symphysis pubis.

From this buffer extend obliquely backward and outward two slots on each side to hold pins and setscrews (under the seat) to fasten the crescent shaped wooden pelvic clamps.

The anciently recognized position of the thighs at right angles with the trunk lessens any lordosis present.[20]

[20] Presented before the Medical and Chirurgical Faculty of Maryland, December 15, 1905.

Jackets are of little or no advantage in high dorsal and cervical caries unless carried around the back of the head and neck, which makes a most bunglesome affair to be worn constantly. Jackets, as a rule, are best adapted to lower dorsal and lumbar diseases, while disease in the upper part of the spine is best treated by the steel brace, which is to be described later on.

The advantages of a plaster jacket are: (1) Its thoroughness and firmness of fixation; it is not uncomfortable as a rule; the surgeon is not dependent on an instrument maker and the appliance stays, as the surgeon leaves it, which is an important consideration where treatment is desired for one of the ignorant classes. (2) The disadvantages of the solid jacket are that it is hot, unclean and may be unsightly and clumsy. It may set up eczema and after a short time comparatively soften and then not fulfill the indications of treatment. When plaster jackets are slit up the front for the applications of lacing, which can be applied by a shoemaker, etc., they offer the disadvantage of being laid aside carelessly by the ignorant who cannot be made to realize the importance of constant support. A good jacket should be of a uniform thickness throughout and not too thick, as was pointed out in speaking of the plaster bandage. It should be well padded with piano felt over all bony points.

UPPER DORSAL AND CERVICAL CASES.

If the disease is above the seventh dorsal vertebra, it should be supplemented by some form of head support; perhaps the most convenient to use in conjunction with a plaster jacket, is the jury mast, which consists of an adjustable steel upright fastened to the middle of the back of the jacket by means of transverse pieces of tin, which can be incorporated in the jacket. The upright follows the contour of the spine and arches as a spring over the back and top of the head and to this can be attached a leather head sling, by means of which more or less head traction and partial suspension may be gained. This, however, is not to be recommended as a reliable method and should only be used as a makeshift.

A second method of removing the superincumbent weight in *cervical caries* is by what is known as the Thomas collar, which consists of a piece of pasteboard, cut out the desired shape to make a full, tall collar, which will rest in front on the sternum and laterally on the shoulders. This pasteboard is thickly and thoroughly padded with oakum, cotton or felt around which are wound ordinary gauze bandages. The patient is allowed to wear this and if it flattens down at all, additional padding can be added until it is of sufficient size to fully extend the neck and take the weight of the head off of the cervical part of the spine. Sometimes, for upper dorsal disease, a steel ring is incorporated in these collars, from which ring extends downward rods terminating in loops. Incorporated in the plaster jacket to be used in this connection are tapes and buckles, by means of which, through the loops, the rods can be forced upward, and thereby additional removal of the superincumbent weight of the head may be effected. This is also a makeshift to be used until a more accurate steel brace is at hand.

THE STEEL BACK BRACE.

For those who can afford it, perhaps one of the cleanest and most efficient spinal supports is to be found in a well fitting steel back brace and apron. This is known as the Taylor back brace, having been devised and modified by Drs. Charles Fayette Taylor and Henry G. Davis, of New York. It is essential, however, that it shall fit as snugly to the skin on either side of the spinous processes from below up to apex of the kyphos. Above this point it should not touch the back so that it will act as a lever. This back brace consists of two parallel uprights from three-eighths inch to one-half inch in width and thick enough and properly tempered to be rigid, which extends over the transverse processes from the fourth lumbar vertebra up to about the third dorsal. All along in the region of disease projecting into the interval between the uprights one-eighth of an inch or more are fastened "steel pressure plates."

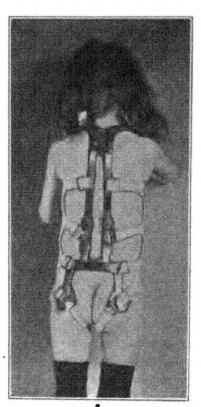

FIG. 57. C. F. TAYLOR'S BACK BRACE.
(Children's Hospital, Boston.)

The uprights are supported at the bottom by a rectangular, two pronged fork, or U-piece, as it is called, the prongs of which are intended to rest in the fossæ, just posterior to the trochanters of the femora. At the top the uprights are joined by a transverse strip of steel. At the top the parallel uprights are bent to an angle of about 45°, as the two oblique pieces pass towards the anterior borders of the trapezius muscle. (Fig. 57.) In front, an apron of twill cotton is made, which is fitted snugly to the patient by means of gores. It extends from the top of the sternum to the symphysis pubis from above downward, and laterally to the mid-axillary lines. This apron is joined to the uprights and forks of the back brace by means of buckles on the latter and straps on the former. For this brace to be efficient, the straps should be kept tight all the time and be non-elastic. In disease above the seventh dorsal vertebra, a single upright should be prolonged from the upper transverse strip of steel on the upper part of this brace to a point on the back of the neck, which corresponds with the atlas. At this point, a hinged ring is attached horizontally, which will encircle the neck and be sufficiently large to support the chin and occiput. At these points, cups of a sufficient size are made of guttapercha or metal to receive the chin and occiput. The single upright, which is

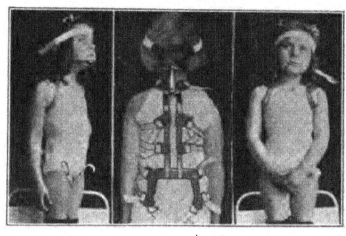

FIG. 59.   FIG. 58.   FIG. 60.

FIG. 58.   C. F. TAYLOR'S BACK BRACE AND HEAD RING (back).
FIG. 59.   C. F. TAYLOR'S BACK BRACE AND HEAD RING (side).   With "apron."
FIG. 60.   C. F. TAYLOR'S BACK BRACE AND HEAD RING (front), with chin piece open and showing the snug fitting apron.

projected from the brace, is adjustable by means of a set-screw to produce any degree of head support. (Figs. 58, 59 and 60.) The ring is detachable by means of a hinge lock at the sides and can be lifted off of the projecting upright. This arrangement is adaptable to cervical, as well as upper dorsal disease. It is sometimes well to have two steel occipital uprights with buckles for fastening a brow band, so that when the chin portion of the ring is opened, as it is necessary to do for the patient to eat, the head will be still supported firmly.

A MODIFICATION OF THE DOLLINGER BRACE FOR CERVICAL AND UPPER DORSAL POTT'S DISEASE.

The well-known Dollinger brace, depicted in Hoffa's text-book, has been familiar to most of us, but, so far as the writer knows, but little employed in this country except by Young. Briefly, it may be likened to a tortoise shell, in which the shell was projected upward or forward, so that the back of the head is also covered. This shell has been made of paper, plaster of paris bandages or felt over the back of a cast of the head, shoulders, back and pelvis of the individual suffering with upper dorsal or cervical Pott's Disease. This shell was reinforced with steel. (Fig. 61.)

During the past two years the writer has employed this device in the treatment of a large number of these cases and can confirm Young's observation, made in 1904, with regard to its value in the treatment of external pachymeningitis, so often a complication of Pott's Disease in this region.

My method of procedure differs from any description I have seen or read of and is as follows: The patient has been hyperextended on the upright kyphotone, or placed on the Brackett hammock, or simply face down on a table, in each case with the thighs at right angles to the trunk to lessen the lower dorsal and lumbar lordosis.

The position obtained by the table method has been found admirable and is the one now most frequently adopted. A strip of stockinet is drawn smoothly over the head, neck, shoulders, and back (or preferably the skin and hair are smeared with vaseline) and semisolid plaster of paris is put on as rapidly as possible before setting; thus, an accurate mold is obtained; or dental wax may be softened in hot water, rolled out into a thin sheet with a bread roller and then molded smoothly over the back of head, neck and trunk. From this a duplicate cast of the patient is obtained in the usual manner by pouring plaster of paris into it.

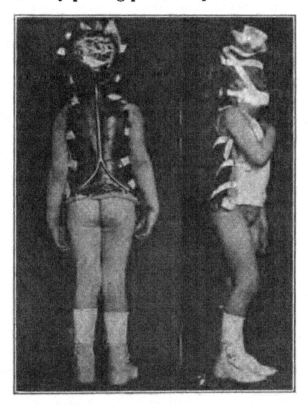

FIG. 61.   MODIFIED DOLLINGER PLASTER OF PARIS SHELL REINFORCED WITH STEEL, AND VARNISHED.

The next step is most important and it is the correction of this cast. First, the shoulders are built upward and backward by additional wet plaster, so that they may be pulled on the patient in these directions by the shell to be made over the cast. The next step is to correct the kyphosis, and this is done by sawing transversely across the cast through the center of the deformity and giving as much hyperextension as one's judgment prompts that the patient will be able to stand and filling in the gap with wet plaster. So far as I know this step was first done by Riely, of my staff. (Fig. 62.)

Now it is a well-known fact that as the kyphosis increases, there is similarly an increase in the lordosis above and below the deformity. Conversely by lessening the lordosis we should, pari passu, lessen the kyphosis. Just as we found hyperextension so valuable in overcoming anatomical, pathological, and mechanical flexion seen in Pott's Disease, which method engrossed us so much in 1894–1895, so of late I have in spinal work (both antero-posterior and lateral) directed my attention to the lordosis and forward tilt of the pelvis,

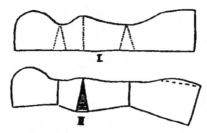

FIG. 62. SHOWING METHOD OF CORRECTING MODEL.

and I feel the correction or lessening of the cervical and lumbar lordosis as important as the dorsal kyphosis.

So the next step is to correct in the cast the lordosis above and below the deformity by sawing a wedge out and mending with wet plaster so that the back is flattened. In the cervical region the object to be striven for is such a position of the head as would correspond with that assumed in endeavoring to make as many "double chins" as possible for thereby the cervical lordosis is lessened to the maximum degree by extreme flexion of the head.

We have observed in children wearing the Taylor back brace and head ring how at times they walk with a forward leaning from the hips which is both ugly and awkward, and

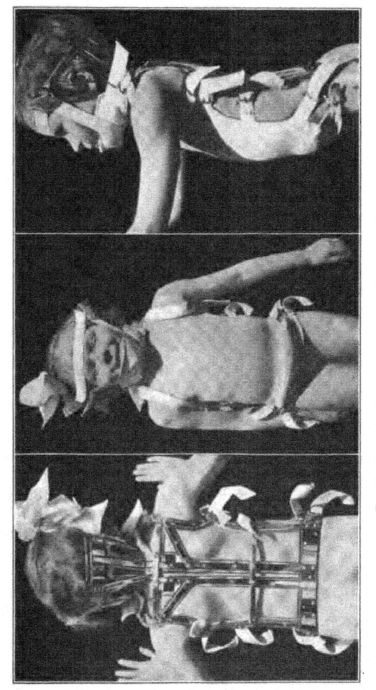

Fig. 63. Author's Modification of the Dollinger Brace.

to help correct this by this method we cut out the cast somewhat in the region of the gluteal muscles. The whole is then smoothed where rough, with draw-knife and sandpaper.

We have now the fully corrected cast ready to make the shell over. It is to be noted that the whole trunk and neck are now longer, by converting the curves into straight lines, which is what we aim for in traction with a head sling. Such a shell is then made over the image of the patient (corrected) and fits admirably.

The objection to the plaster of paris, paper or felt shells is that they so soon soften, especially at the shoulders, and as the shoulder portion is of one of the most essential parts, it is a serious objection. These shells take a great deal of care and time to make of felt and of a uniform thickness throughout of plaster of paris, so that they must necessarily be expensive, and if of short life, the parents of patients rebel, and are not satisfactory to the surgeon in obtaining reliable results.

Therefore I am now using the corrected cast as in the modified Dollinger brace, but have no shell, and instead the outlines are of steel with two steel uprights as in the C. F. Taylor back brace, a transverse pelvic piece below the posterior superior spines, and extending downward and forward to within an inch of the anterior superior spines. The shoulder and neck outline is of steel and the head portion is like a truncated Dollinger brace which we have used in plaster also, feeling that the portion corresponding with the posterior part of the parietals was superfluous and only the occipital and temporals required support.[30] (Fig. 63.)

Instead of a steel circle or U-piece to support the back of the head, Riely suggested a continuation forward from the top of the lateral steel rods just above the ears to the anterior hair margin, and on the ends were placed two

[30] R. T. Taylor: American Journal Orthopædic Surgery, April, 1906.

buckles to pull more vertically upward on the chin sling and hold the brow band. This brow band does not slip.

The uprights corresponding to the C. F. Taylor brace are placed as close as possible to the spinous processes, thus avoiding the posterior superior spinous processes of the ilia and instead of the pressure plates in the region of disease being inside, project half an inch or more on the outside of the uprights, thus affording better support to the entire region of the transverse processes and ribs.

The region of the head, neck, shoulders and deformity can be filled in partially or entirely either with stiff leather or woven copper, or aluminum wire, or left open. It is never necessary to have the remainder thus covered. All uprights on the skin side have cemented on a layer of leather, then kid. If the plaster shells are used we line them throughout with one piece of piano felt, which is cemented to the plaster with shellac, but this is hot and soon has an odor.

Nothing gave one of my recumbent adult patients, who was suffering with both sensory and motor sarcomatous paralysis and intense hyperæsthesia and cramps, the comfort afforded by a steel reinforced plaster shell made over such a corrected cast as described, for thereby firmer fixation, traction, hyperextension, and hyperflexion were secured than I had been able to supply *by any other means* of traction, fixation and hyperextension.

It is needless to say that these braces are completed by an apron, such as is worn with the C. F. Taylor back brace, a brow band, chin sling, and neck band, which latter helps to lessen the cervical lordosis.

The advantages of this steel brace are rigidity, durability and lightness. It gives support where it is most needed, not only over the transverse processes in the region of the disease but over the ribs and shoulders. It is made over a cast corrected in accordance with the therapeutic requirements from pathological findings and must fit. It is easily adjusted and one can see whether pressure and support are exerted in the proper places, which is impossible with the Dollinger or similar modified braces. For patients living at a distance who cannot return for brace adjustment this brace will be found very serviceable, for once fitted it is so rigid it is not likely to change its shape, as I have found is often the case with the C. F. Taylor back brace.

| The Goldthwait collar is a very useful brace in many cases of cervical disease and consists of a cup for the chin and one for the occiput, supported on a ring, which is attached on either side of the neck by means of steel wire uprights, which in turn are attached to a piece of steel, which passes from the bottom of the ribs on one side up over the shoulders around on the sternum, and up over the opposite shoulder down to the other side. A single strap will hold these uprights in place in passing around the thorax. A hinge and lock are provided as in the C. F. Taylor head ring.   (Fig. 64.)

Appliances are faulty from (1) flexibility; (2) imperfect fixation from a bad fitting brace, loose or elastic straps. Axillary crutch supports attached to a steel waist band afford a variable and unreliable support, especially in children whose hips are not large and are ridiculous as supporting the shoulders and not the spine. They should not be bought or sold having no scientific basis in Potts' Disease.

VACCINES AND THE OPSONIC INDEX.

Much interest has been revived of late by the work of Sir Almroth Wright,[31] in an endeavor to get a definite index by clinical blood examination of the degree of immunity possessed by patients in various diseases. Results at measur-

[31] Proceedings of the Royal Society, No. 72, Oct. 31, 1903; No. 73, March 7, 1904; No. 74, Sept. 28, 1904, and Jan., 1905. Bulloch: Practitioner, Dec., 1905, and Lancet, 1905, ii, 1605. Wright: Roy. Soc. Proc., vol. 71, 1902. Lancet, July 5, 1902. Leishman: British Med. Jour., Jan. 11, 1902.

ing this degree of immunity or increased resistance had not been satisfactory with agglutinins and bacteriolysins, so that Wright suggested that there must be some substance in the serum which, when combined with the white corpuscles (polynuclear leucocytes or phagocytes) would show in varying conditions a varying degree of phagocytosis or power of ingesting the invading bacteria. He thus, in a way combined Metchnikoff's theory of phagocytosis with Ehrlich's "side chain" theory of the action of the serum. This substance in the serum he called opsonin, which means "to prepare a meal for." Further, he showed that this amount of opsonin could be increased or diminished by the hypodermic injection in definite doses of emulsions or "vaccines" of the infecting bacteria destroyed by heat. The comparison of the action of the serum of the patient with the serum or a "pool" of the sera of several normal persons, he called the "opsonic index."

For example, if 100 phagocytes combined with the normal serum ate on an average 6 bacteria each, which he would call normal or 1, and the same number of phagocytes of the patient gave only an average of 4, he would compute the opsonic index of that patient by the proportion 6 : 1:: 4 : x or x would equal 0.66 in this particular example. If the index was subnormal, the power of resistance or degree of immunity was called low and if above normal, high.

In an infected individual, however, this index is variable and may possibly be low one day, high the next and on the normal line the third day, so this variability must be taken into consideration in an infected individual, even without artificial vaccination, and is a valuable point in diagnosis. Possibly an autovaccination, as Wright pointed out, may or may not take place from the seat of the infection by massage or movement and cause this over- or under-stimulation in opsonic production in the patient.

We know clinically by laboratory examinations on this point that too large dosage of vaccine, or vaccinations given at too frequent intervals, will lower the opsonic index, and moderate and proper doses will raise it. In other words you cannot unduly push this production of the opsonic substance in the patient's serum.

Briefly, Wright's technique[32] as pursued by Dr. E. A. Knorr and the writer in our observations is as follows:

1. A small tube is used to collect 15 to 20 drops of the patient's blood from the finger or ear and a similar tube to collect blood from a normal individual or individuals. These tubes are put in a water or electric centrifugal machine, until all the corpuscles are driven down, leaving the clear supernatant *serum* above.

2. *Blood* is drawn from the finger or ear of a normal individual into a small test tube containing an aqueous solution of 1 per cent sodium chloride and 1.5 per cent sodium citrate (or .1 per cent ammonium oxalate) to prevent clotting until the solution is a bright red, then centrifugalize. Pipette off the solution above the corpuscles which have been thrown down. Fill the test tube with 1.5 per cent sodium chloride solution, shake well to wash corpuscles free of serum and again centrifugalize and pipette off the supernatant fluid. This leaves the lighter white corpuscles as the "cream" on top of the red corpuscles.

3. A *bacterial emulsion* must be prepared to mix with the serum and white corpuscles. In the case of the tubercle bacillus, take a small quantity, about the size of a grain of rice, of the dried preferably fatty or heated sterile tubercle bacillus powder of Von Rook, Burroughs, Wellcome & Co. or Trudeau and mix it in a smooth agate mortar with a few drops of .1 per cent. salt solution, adding drop by drop additional salt solution, until a uniform solution like very

[32] Simon's modification.

thin milk is obtained. Centrifugalize this and retain all the supernatant fluid as the "tubercular emulsion," the clumps to which the tubercle bacillus is prone having been thrown down.

The staphylococcus or similar emulsion is made by taking a oese full of a 24 hour agar culture mixing it with 5 cc. of sterile salt solution and then centrifugalizing and retaining the supernatant fluid containing them, as the staphylococcus, etc., emulsion.

The next step is to mix these with the sera and corpuscles. First, long capillary pipettes are drawn out in the Bunsen burner and a teat is put on the large end. With a glass marking pencil an inch or two is marked off on the capillary end and the normal serum is drawn up to this mark, then a bubble is allowed to enter and the same quantity of the bacterial emulsion is drawn in. Finally another bubble is admitted and from the cream of the corpuscles the same quantity is drawn in of the leucocytes.

These three are then squirted out on a glass slide or watch crystal, thoroughly mixed, drawn into the capillary, squirted out again and mixed and again drawn in some distance into the capillary, which is then sealed in the flame of the Bunsen burner, the teat taken off and the pipette labeled with the glass marking pencil. The same procedure is then gone through with all the sera from the patients.

If more than one bacterium is under investigation a normal or pool or control mixture must be made of the normal serum, bacterial emulsion and leucocytes in each case as the tubercle control would not do for determining a coccus opsonic index, it goes without saying and vice versa.

These labeled pipettes are then put flat in the thermostat for 15 minutes at 37 degrees C., when the closed end is broken, the teat is put on again and the mixture squirted on one end of a slide; with the end of another slide the smear is made and it is air dried.

In the case of cocci the slide is fixed by very gentle warming over the Bunsen burner, testing frequently with the hand that it be not overheated and this method is preferable to alcohol hardening as the cocci are shriveled thereby. Very frequently, if thoroughly air dried, fixation by heat is unnecessary.[33] It is then stained with 1 per cent aqueous solution of methylene blue.

With tubercle bacilli fix the air dried slide in a saturated solution of bichloride of mercury two minutes, wash, stain with carbo-fuchsin, boil gently over flame, being careful the slide is always covered with the staining solution and no drying or precipitation occurs, which can be accomplished by means of a pipette end and not overheating. Decolorize rapidly in 2 per cent solution of sulphuric acid, wash and neutralize the acid in a .1 per cent carbonate of soda solution, wash and counter stain with one per cent aqueous solution of methylene blue, and wash thoroughly.

When air dried the slide is ready to count. This we did with a mechanical stage and counted in nearly all instances 200 polynuclear leucocytes. We used two indexes, Wright's, which requires counting the individual bacteria ingested in each leucocyte and Simon's, which calls for the percentage number of phagocyting leucocytes and is accurate, perhaps more so than Wright's, if the bacteria tend to clump and is much easier on the eyes. Both indices show identical variations but Wright's, if very high, shows a much higher curve than Simon's, which is not open to the error introduced by the ingestion of clumps of bacteria notably the tubercle bacilli which seriously affect Wright's index. In many instances we made both counts.[34]

The following is a characteristic chart of an acute tubercular osteitis of the cervical vertebræ with proper vac-

[33] Knorr.
[34] Simon, Lamar and Bispham: Jour. Experimental Med., Dec. 21, 1906.

cination and excessive vaccination.   There was no temperature reaction nor reactionary symptoms of any kind.   The
patient was in bed with head traction and the symptoms
seemed to abate perhaps more rapidly with the vaccination.

Koch's tuberculin T. R. was employed in beginning doses
of $\frac{1}{5000}$ mgm. and increased to $\frac{1}{100}$ mgm.

A characteristic secondarily infected case of lumbar
Potts' Disease, cultures from sinuses showing staphylococ-

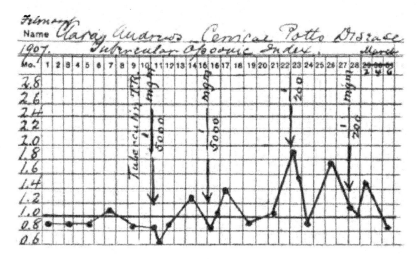

CHART A. TUBERCULAR OPSONIC INDICES.
Arrows indicate vaccinations.

cus, gave the following chart after vaccination with very
appreciable lessening of the discharge, which had continued
for months with hectic fever, which also abated.   One billion staphylococci were given as the initial dose, one billion
three hundred million as the second and two billion as the
third dose with a week's interval between each.   The staphylococcus vaccine is prepared by adding 10 cc. of 1.5 per cent
salt solution (sterile) to a 24 hour smear agar culture of the
aureus, thoroughly oscillating, then pouring on a second
similar tube and so on until four tubes have the cocci thus

washed off. Equal quantities of freshly drawn blood in a
pipette is mixed with this suspension and a count made in
comparison with the red cells on a slide. Thus we can
determine in a given volume how many cocci we have.
The vaccine is then boiled in a sterile tube for thirty minutes and 0.25 per cent lysol added as a preservative. It is
then incubated twenty-four hours and cultures made to be
sure it is sterile.

CHART B. STAPHYLOCOCCUS OPSONIC INDICES.

We were thus able to confirm in these and many other
charts, Wright's observation, that in infected cases, we
have a high, low and variable index for that organism.

As yet we have not been able to get our cases up to a high
level of immunity, as shown by the opsonic index and have
them remain at that level.

The opsonic index seems a most valuable guide as to
proper dosage of vaccines, which we cannot observe, otherwise clinically finely, unless we give so much a temperature
reaction is produced, which is to be avoided.

Wright advises vaccination when the index is near 1,
that is, neither when high nor low or when rising.

In normal serum the opsonic power is destroyed by heating to 60 degrees C. for ten minutes, and this does not occur in diseased conditions and the serum is called "immune serum," so that phagocytosis occurs almost as readily after heating as before, which is not the case (*i. e.*, phagocytosis) with heated normal serum. This is a possible means of diagnosis.

TREATMENT OF COMPLICATIONS.

I. *Treatment of Cold Abscess.*

1. Expectant treatment often yields good results and as long as the general health keeps good, or does not suffer, the abscesses should not be opened unless pressure symptoms are manifest, such as interference with any of the respiratory or digestive functions, pressure on the bowels or blood vessels, or on a nerve or seem in danger of secondary infection through the skin and the blood examination gives a high leucocyte count. If the skin becomes very thin over such an abscess, so as to be nothing more than what we might term a paper covering, the abscess may be opened to save the bedclothes, as it is practically impossible to get at the seat of the disease, and remove all the tuberculous material and focus which is producing the contents of the abscess. In all cases they should be sewed up after three or four days of drainage unless secondarily infected, as they are most prone to infection by the pyogenic cocci, which the patient gives evidence of by "hectic fever." In which case the patient will probably have a discharging sinus which will continue as long as the disease is active, and may interfere with the application of a proper support. It should be borne in mind that these are "cold abscesses" and simply consist of broken down bone and caseous material. As a rule, they are surrounded by a thick, fibrous wall of granulation tissue, so that absorption must, of a necessity, take place very slowly, and the general health suffer therefrom proportion-

ately very little. An abscess may be the size of a large orange or even bigger, and yet it is better to leave it alone unless some dangerous symptom appears. If opened simple incision and evacuation yields better results than when extensive curetting is employed—as is done in acute ab-

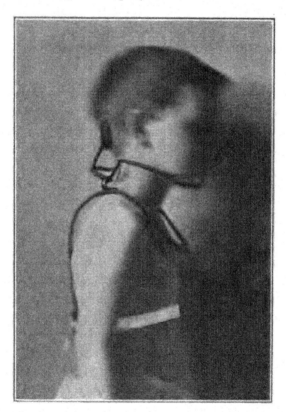

FIG. 64. THE GOLDTHWAIT COLLAR.

scesses. Subcutaneous silver wire sutures should be put in at once and the edges approximated immediately or in a very few days after evacuation in an endeavor to obtain primary union. Many large abscesses are entirely absorbed.

2. Frequent aspiration, with the idea of promoting absorption, is of questionable value, as many of the products

of the abscess cannot be withdrawn through an aspirating needle of small or medium size or trocar.

3. The injection of fluids or antiseptics to promote absorption or resolution has not been very satisfactory; however, where a sinus exists, it should be injected thoroughly and washed out occasionally with peroxide of hydrogen, and after this injected with a 10 per cent solution of iodoform in olive oil, or better, as we have found, with 2½ per cent solution of the 40 per cent formalin stock solution. If there is no secondary infection, sterile water or decinormal salt solution or *dry mopping* out with gauze is preferable.

4. *Incision.* The indications for incision are (1) definite localization of the abscess; (2) pressure symptoms of a disturbing nature, and (3) the possibility of easy and perfect drainage, flushing thoroughly with hot sterile water when the incision is to be dried, sutured and the walls of the cavity approximated by compresses and tight bandages.

The writer is distinctly opposed to the necessarily blind efforts at curetting the vertebral bodies, for the traumatism of healthy tissues leads to extension and not removal of the disease with the production of septic sinuses, which last for years and result in amyloid disease and death often.

II. *Treatment of Psoas Contraction.*

1. Fixation on a bedframe is indicated. An inclined plane which can be gradually lowered is to be used to support the drawn leg, and weight and pulley traction by means of Buck's extension usually overcome the trouble when of recent origin. Traction is to be made in the line of the deformity. (Fig. 9.)

2. In old neglected cases, anæsthesia with forcible correction may break up any fibrous adhesions and stretch the shortened muscles (psoas and iliacus). But this procedure is rarely the one to choose. "Brisement forcé" it is called.

3. Tenotomy or myotomy of the tensor vaginæ femoris, long head of the rectus and sartorius muscles may be necessary.

4. But, preferably, subtrochanteric osteotomy must be employed (Gant's operation) in resistant cases. This consists of dividing the femur just below the intertrochanteric line with an osteotome and mallet, which operation will be spoken of more at length under hip disease.

III. *Treatment of Paralysis.*

1. Mechanical treatment is to be employed in all cases with recumbency, fixation, hyperextension and perhaps extension by means of weights attached to the head and legs. This is the best and most reliable mode of treatment.

2. Of the medicinal remedies, the iodide of potassium in increasing and large doses, and ergot and the application of the cautery over the diseased area, have been recommended, but are of little value without thorough fixation.

3. Hyperextension (forcible) by the kyphotone or some of the other methods mentioned of applying a jacket have yielded good results at times. Occasionally sufficiently thorough bed fixation is not obtainable and a jacket should be worn in recumbency as well.

4. Laminectomy should be done when the pressure symptoms do not improve under the prolonged treatment after a year or more of recumbency and fixation, but it is a most unwise procedure if avoidable, as the bodies of the vertebræ offer no support and if the laminæ are removed there is only the support of articular processes. Paralysis may then recur. (Painter.)

5. Costo-transversectomy or the removal of an inch or two of the rib and transverse process at the seat of the disease on one side and then puncturing the abscess cavity in the vertebral body by the finger, a probe or curette yields

satisfactory results in prolonged cases and should be tried before laminectomy is resorted to.

TREATMENT IN GENERAL.

Treatment in general should aim at obtaining for each case (1) the most nourishing food; (2) fresh air ;(3) exercise; (4) tonics, such as strychnin, cod liver oil and iron especially.

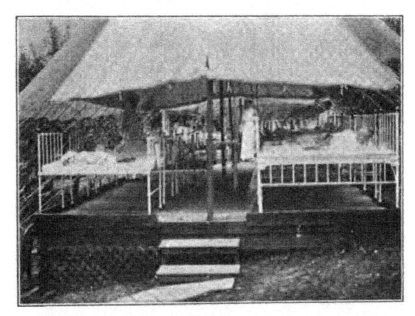

FIG. 65. A TENT WARD AT THE MOUNTAIN HOSPITAL FOR SURGICAL TUBERCULOSIS.

(Established in 1897 at Blue Ridge Summit, Pa., as a branch of the Baltimore Hospital for Crippled Children.)

Preparations of beef blood are helpful in the anæmia of amyloid cases. In other words, in these cases the general treatment should be what we would give a case with tubercular disease elsewhere. Many cases are much benefited by residence in a high altitude, as is the case in consumption, with out-of-door life and our cases which have four or five

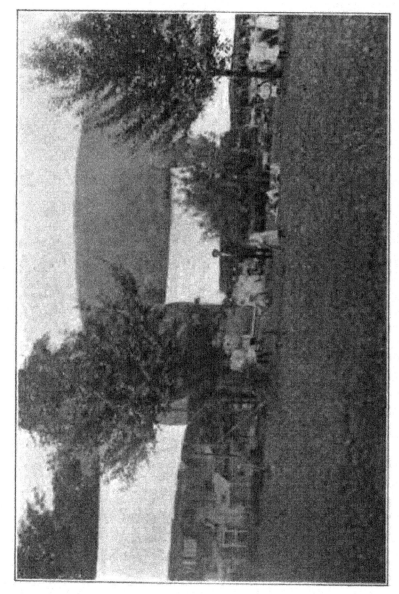

FIG. 86. SHOWING PORTIONS OF THREE TENT WARDS AT THE MOUNTAIN HOSPITAL.

months at the mountain hospital in the summer, all show
the benefit in the fall.   This we have insisted on since 1897.
(Figs. 65 and 66.)   The vaccines certainly seem helpful.

It is needless to say that the great aim of each surgeon
called upon to treat a case of Pott's Disease should be to

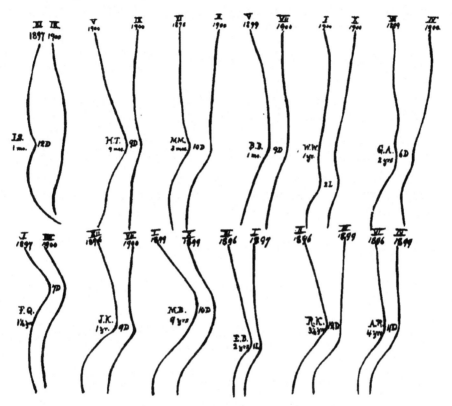

FIG. 67. THE DURATION OF THE DISEASE WHEN FIRST SEEN IS INDICATED ON
THE LEFT OF THE DEFORMITY, TRACINGS OF SOME LOWER DORSAL AND LUMBAR
CASES OF POTT'S DISEASE, SHOWING RESULTS OF TREATMENT, BY PLASTER OF
PARIS JACKETS.

make his diagnosis as soon as possible and institute the most
thorough means of persistent immobilization and hyperextension *early*, to prevent the increase or the production
of this dreadful and disfiguring deformity.   There is no

question that the responsibility for severe deformity in such cases, of which we see evidences constantly, rests on the family physician, who by ignorance or halfway measures of his own or by attempting to shirk his duty to his patient in referring him to unskilled instrument-makers, whose pathology is an unknown quantity, reaps his reward in seeing his patient gradually become deformed.

An exception to this anathema is the folly sometimes found in parents, who will not carry out the prescribed treatment to the letter.

Records of Cases. When the patient is first seen the lead tape should be molded along the spinous processes to show any deviation from the normal. The molded tape is then laid edgewise and used as a ruler on the patient's history and with a pencil a record curve is made. At each subsequent visit a similar tracing is made so that the efficacy of the treatment in preventing the increase of the deformity may be observed and more rigid methods employed if necessary. (Fig. 67.)

CHAPTER VI.

NON-TUBERCULOUS DISEASES OR AFFECTIONS OF THE SPINE.

1. *Rachitic Kyphosis.*

Frequently in rickety infants before the third year, one sees a marked angular spinal deformity, which may be mistaken for Pott's Disease in the dorso-lumbar region, with lordosis in the cervical and upper dorsal region. The diagnosis is not difficult if one bears in mind the other symptoms of rachitis, viz: the square head, beaded ribs, enlarged radial epiphyses, prominent abdomen, Harrison's groove, bent extremities, etc.

If one places the child on the face and the deformity is of short duration the curve can be flattened by pressing with the palm of the left hand, while with the right the child's legs are raised to produce hyperextension of the spine. It should be kept recumbent on its back on a frame until the acute symptoms of rickets disappear. If of long duration, massage should be given morning and evening to the spinal muscles and hyperextension employed by means of a padded block on the Bradford frame, as indicated under Pott's Disease. In either case recumbency is indicated, together with good hygienic treatment, such as cold sponging, proper food and tonics, to be spoken of later more in detail under rickets. (Fig. 68.)

At times it is advisable to put the child on a kyphotone and apply a plaster jacket, made to lace preferably, or an antero-posterior brace to be described under Section 14 of this chapter may be employed.

If the rachitic kyphosis is allowed to persist we may have when the child walks or stands the "rachitic attitude" with exaggeration of the dorsal kyphosis and lumbar lordosis as a result of muscular relaxation and forward tilting of the pelvis. (Fig. 69.) Or if the infantile kyphosis is more of the lumbar type the dorsal curve may become compensatorily less marked with the resulting "flat back."

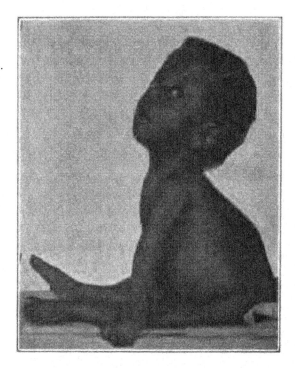

FIG. 68. RACHITIC DORSO-LUMBAR KYPHOSIS.

Lateral curvature of the spine may be a sequela of untreated rachitic kyphosis from the habitual faulty attitude and weakness together with lateral body bending or twisting of the spine or pelvis during the period of softening of the bones.

2. *Typhoid Spine.*

Gibney[35] first described a spinal disease, simulating Pott's Disease, but without deformity, which followed typhoid fever, or occurred during its course, in which the articulations or perispondylitic structures become secondarily affected. It is characterized by pain, weakness and stiffness. The diagnosis is clear from the history of the febrile attack and relief is afforded by recumbency, opiates, the Paquelin cautery, massage and later a spinal brace. Osler, Keen, Park, Quincke and others have reported cases.[36]

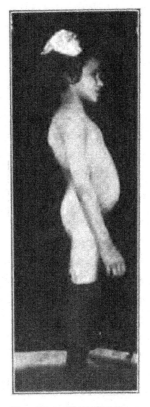

FIG. 69. THE RACHITIC ATTITUDE. "ROUND-HOLLOW BACK."

3. *Scarlet Fever Periostitis and "Gonorrhœal Rheumatism" of the Spine.*

These troubles are rare and result in pathological changes and symptoms, which resemble typhoid spine. Gonorrhœa often results in stiffness of the spine from adhesive ankylosis or proliferative exostoses and some consider it one of the causes of rheumatoid arthritis of the spine, usually spoken of as spondylitis deformans, to be discussed under that heading later (Section 6). Much benefit may result from a sterile emulsion of gonococci as a vaccine, to be spoken of further on in diseases of the extremities.

[35] Trans., Amer. Orth. Assoc., vols. ii and iv.
[36] Johns Hopkins Hospital Reports, iv, 80.

Locally the treatment is the same as in typhoid spine, the plaster of paris jacket often affording great relief.

4. *Syphilitic Disease of the Spine.*

In children specific bone disease may be inherited or in older patients be acquired, but one rarely finds gummatous lesions in the spine, the long bones showing oftener the characteristic periostitis or osteochondritis at epiphyseal and diaphyseal junctions. Should the spine become secondarily involved the symptoms and treatment would be the same as those found under tuberculosis, with the addition of the therapeutic measures demanded for lues. Of course, it is possible to imagine tuberculous osteitis of the vertebræ and syphilitic lesions elsewhere, but Bradford and Lovett[37] rather doubt a primary specific osseous manifestation in the spine.

5. *Acute Arthritis of the Occipito-Atlantoid Articulation.*

Whitman calls attention to this affection which may follow tonsillitis, diphtheria or other contagious diseases infecting the pharynx by extension. It resembles a localized rheumatism and can be distinguished from tuberculous disease by the acute onset and from acute torticollis by the fact that all motions are restricted and not simply those controlled by the sterno-cleido-mastoid and trapezius.

The treatment should consist of the local treatment of the causative disease in the fauces and pharynx and a fixative support in recumbency by means of sandbags. This should be followed later by massage and manipulations to overcome the subsequent stiffness.

6. *Spondylitis Deformans.*

Synonyms. Osteo-arthritis of the spine; ankylosis of the spine; rheumatism of the spine; and rheumatoid arthritis of

[37] 2d ed., p. 155.

the spine; spondylose rhizomélique of Marie. (When all joints are involved this constitutes the "ossified man" of the museums.)

Pathology. There is a chronic ankylosing inflammation affecting primarily the ossification of ligaments and prevertebral coverings of the spine, a form of ossifying periostitis, which binds the vertebræ firmly together. It may be limited to a few vertebræ, to one region or include the whole

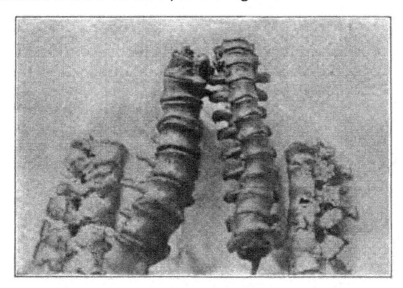

Fig. 70. Spondylitis Deformans, Showing Osteophytes on Either Side and Scoliotic Vertebræ in Center.

spine and the articulations with the ribs. It may be a part of a general rheumatoid arthritis involving other joints, but under the name spondylitis deformans the spine alone is understood to be involved and there is a proliferation of bone in this region as exostoses. It may be a sequela of acute inflammatory rheumatism, traumatism, gonorrhœa in young male adults or other infections but is more common in women past middle life. According to Nichols of Harvard the causes are various and the different types are simply different stages of the same process.   (Fig. 70.)

Symptoms. Stiffness of the spine follows an acute onset and gradually increases. Muscular spasm, headache as of a "steel band around the brow," weakness in the extremities (more often in the arms) and radiating, peripheral pain from pressure on nerve roots as they emerge from the spinal cord may extend to arms or legs depending on the region involved. Neurasthenic symptoms are characteristic.

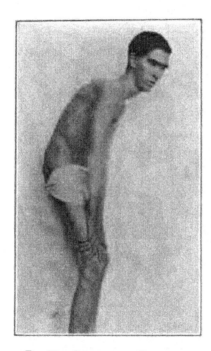

FIG. 71. SPONDYLITIS DEFORMANS.
(Showing Maximum Degree of Extension.)

Any region or all regions of the spine may be involved. At times the muscular spasm in cervical disease with spasmodic head movements or "dragging" as it is called by the patient is a most distressing symptom, until relieved by an ankylosis or subsidence of the symptoms of inflammation. Distinct localized swelling is sometimes present and palpable or even visible over the transverse and spinous processes. A strenuous, nervous life, overwork, ill health, or privations in food and comforts will be found to play a part in the ætiology.

Some patients describe the muscular spasm giving a sensation in cervical disease as if they "were horses in check reins" and are constantly moving the head as much as possible in the effort to relieve this tension and spasm in the trapezius and deeper muscles. Some have "pain across the shoulders as though carrying an iron bar" and some weakness in legs. Nearly all these cases are neurotic, irritable and high-strung from the prolonged suffering. The duration of the disease usually covers several years and is chronic. The pain fortunately stops after a time, but is of course relieved sooner by treatment. There is no angular deformity as in Pott's Disease, but the

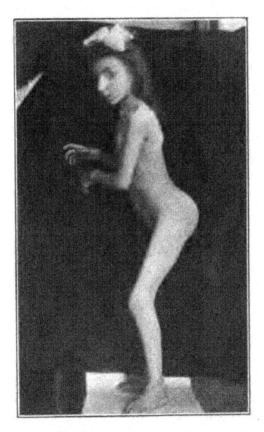

FIG. 72. GENERAL RHEUMATOID ARTHRITIS INVOLVING SPINE ALSO.

whole spine with ribs may become ankylosed and bowed concavely forward. The cervical spine is usually ankylosed last of all. Breathing is abdominal when ankylosis occurs between the dorsal vertebræ and the ribs. (Fig. 71.)

Treatment. Tonics, such as cod liver oil, strychnin or iron should be given. Rest of the part in the acute stage is of the first importance. Of local remedies, the Paquelin cautery, self-suspension by the head sling, recumbency with head traction, the Thomas collar or steel head support, a back brace or plaster jacket afford. most relief during the acute stage. Especially if pain is increased on motion, a brace will relieve the muscular spasm and prevent deformity. Rubber heels lessen the jar on the spine in the acute period. Massage and Swedish movements are only helpful later and intensify the trouble in the early stages.

7. *Osteitis Deformans or Paget's Disease.*

This disease was first described by Paget in 1877[38] and hence bears his name. It is a chronic affection of the bones, characterized by kyphosis of the spine and hypertrophy and softening of the bones, and those bearing weight become unnaturally curved and misshapen. (Fig. 73.)

Pathology. A section of an affected bone shows it to be markedly increased in size and somewhat in length by a combination of internal osteoporosis and a formative osteitis under the periosteum.

This disease occurs in adult life and chiefly in old age, is rarely in one bone but usually is symmetrical and general in its distribution. The spine is kyphotic, as before stated, the head enormously enlarged and the arms and legs are bowed. Pain is rarely present and then of a subacute rheumatic type. There are no marked symptoms. The ætiology is unknown and treatment is palliative by means of braces to prevent the bending of the spine and legs; a C. F. Taylor back brace is to be used for the former and supporting braces for the latter (to be described in detail under infantile paralysis).

[38] Med. Chir. Trans., 1877, vol. xl, and 1882, lxv.

8. *Cancer of the Spine.*

Primary malignant bony growths in the spine are remarkably unusual in children. However sarcoma is more often seen than carcinoma and when found other portions of the body will have first shown evidences of the disease.

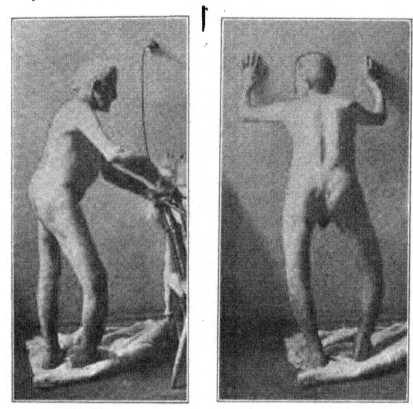

FIG. 73.   PAGET'S DISEASE WITH LONG CERVICO-DORSO-LUMBAR KYPHOSIS.
(Courtesy of Dr A. D. Atkinson.)

If present in the spine, the symptoms are severe as elsewhere, the pain and paralysis from pressure on the nerves and cord are constantly present, the course is rapid, the cachexia as shown by the general appearance, anæmia and systemic depression is noticeable. Early dissolution may be anticipated. No remedies save anodynes are of service, and mechanical appliances are helpful if fixation is perfect, in the relief of pain, and the kyphosis, so characteristic in tuberculosis of the spine, is not present; one rather finds in

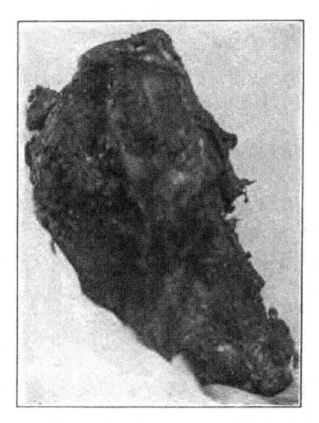

FIG. 74. OSTEO-SARCOMA OF THE SPINE. FOURTH TO EIGHTH DORSAL VERTEBRAL BODIES AND ADJACENT RIBS INVOLVED. LITTLE OR NO POSTERIOR CURVATURE.

lumbar disease on palpation in the abdomen the large growth. If the contour of the spine is changed posteriorly it is rather as a rounded tumor mass than as an acute angular curvature. (Fig. 74.)·

9. *Traumatisms to the Spine.*

Severe sprains, slight or severe fractures of the spine may occur, especially in the cervical region as from diving accidents, but recumbency and supports together with head traction in bed will clear up the diagnosis of traumatic cases in a comparatively short time, especially when taken in conjunction with the history of immediate onset of the trouble after an accident, in contradistinction to the gradual onset in tuberculous disease.

Fracture in the dorsal region, according to Kummel[39] with symptoms of pain and weakness may result in a rounded angular deformity like Pott's Disease, which in untreated cases may increase and persist indefinitely, from a rarefying osteitis.

Compression or impacted fractures of the vertebral bodies without deformity may occur as the result of falls from a height and Painter[40] has reported cases of traumatic rupture of the posterior spinous ligaments producing a deformity similar to Pott's Disease.

Diagnosis as to the nature of the trouble is to be made by a careful review of the history and examination of the case, with, if possible, the aid of the X-ray.

Treatment. Fixation in plaster of paris in cases of fracture or recumbency with head and leg traction, so often omitted, must be used. In the early cases approximation of the fragments if obtainable is to be tried for. Some form of cervical or spinal support is to be used until all symptoms of weakness disappear. Wiring the spinous processes together has also been employed.

Pressure symptoms on the cord are to be relieved if due to bony spiculæ by their removal by operative measures when other means fail, but in all cases spinal immobilization

[39] Deutsche Med. Wochens.. 1895, N. 11.
[40] Transactions, Amer. Orthopædic Assoc.

is essential. Massage is useful later, as in fractures elsewhere, to restore function as far as possible.

10. *Acute Osteomyelitis of the Spine.*

This is an uncommon disease, occurring usually in young
adults in the lumbar region and less than 50 cases are recorded.[a]   Like all acute inflammations, its onset is sudden
with chill or convulsion, fever, marked pain, tenderness over
the spine (unlike Pott's Disease) and pyæmic constitutional
symptoms. A typhoidal condition frequently supervenes.
Abscess and paralysis are common complications but the
former may extend in an anterior direction and escape detection. Large vertebral sequestra may result from the bone
necrosis. The death rate is stated at about 60 per cent.
The streptococcus or staphylococcus are usually responsible. Cases involving the spinous or transverse processes
show much less severe symptoms and are more accessible
for treatment.

Treatment. Necessarily immediate incision is indicated
with the subsequent treatment given all acute abscesses,
and the spine is to be supported in recumbency by a jacket
or brace during the rapid formation of new bone to prevent
distortion, but angular curvatures similar to Pott's Disease
rarely result from this cause.

11. *The Neurotic or Hysterical Spine.*
"Railroad Spine."

This condition is more common in female adults of the
nervous or neurasthenic type, but in some instances the
symptoms appear to be the direct result of slight injuries.

[a] Hahn: Beiträge zur Klin. Chir., Bd. 45, H. 1, 899; Müller: Deutsche Zeitschrift
für Chir., Bd. 41; Makins and Abbott: Amer. Surg., May, 1896; Chipault: Gaz. des
Hôp., 1897, lxx, 1442; Riese: Centralbl. für Chir., 1898, S. 585; Tixier: Bulletin
Med., June, 1895.

There may be no deformity, but usually there is a drooping of the shoulders, from general atony.

One of the chief characteristics is the extreme local tenderness (which we do not see in Pott's Disease) in a certain region of the spine more commonly at or near the vertebra prominens. This is easily detected by palpation and it will be found that the skin is said to be hyperæsthetic at these definite points. There is no pain at the peripheral distribution of the nerves as in tuberculous kyphosis. They suffer much with backache and tire easily.

The treatment should include tonics, general attention to hygiene, rest, the cautery for its mental effect, massage to the weak region and a spinal support if necessary. Other cases require vigorous gymnastics.

12. "Backache."

This may be a condition associated with lordosis in overworked and pregnant women, requiring treatment. It is also found often in badly deformed cases of hunchback and coxalgia, with marked flexion and adduction deformity of the legs, associated with lordosis.

Treatment. The acute stage is best treated by recumbency, massage and the cautery, followed by strapping of the back with intersecting strips of adhesive plaster. The belladonna plaster used so frequently by the laity may afford this supporting treatment, as well as having its anæsthetic effect on the pain.

Some light form of steel brace or plaster jacket may be necessary. For a pendulous abdomen, an abdominal supporting bandage and perineal straps put on in recumbency, with the pelvis raised, is essential in the atonic with a tendency to enteroptosis, but should be supplemented with leg and body raising exercises and massage to prevent further muscular atrophy.

13. *Spondylolisthesis.*

This is a condition first described by Killian in 1854 and more thoroughly investigated by Neugebauer in 1890, in which one of the bodies of the lumbar vertebræ, usually the fourth or fifth, slip forward and downward, making the brim of the pelvis narrower antero-posteriorly than it should

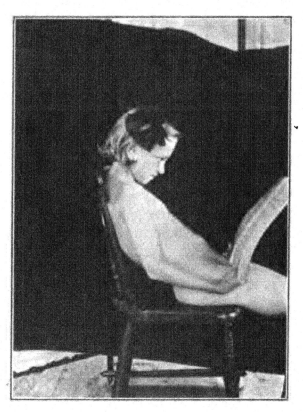

FIG. 75. ONE CAUSE OF KYPHOSIS, "LYING DOWN IN CHAIRS."

be normally. It is therefore chiefly important from an obstetrical standpoint. Lordosis is increased, but the spinous processes are not depressed, as one would suppose, but the laminæ seem stretched, elongated or separated. It may be due to disease, injury or congenital malformation.   The pain if present is best relieved by a plaster jacket or brace.[47]

14. *Antero-posterior Curvatures of the Spine.*

Under these we have the long curves involving the whole spine in the kyphosis seen in infancy (when the baby cannot

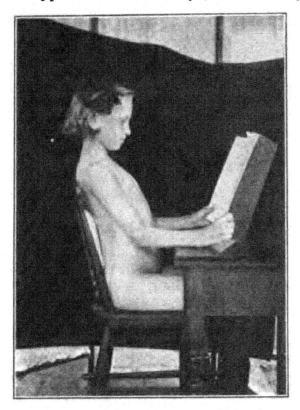

FIG. 76. THE PROPER SITTING POSITION.

hold the head up), in old age and after acute illnesses, and as a sign of weakness.   When a child grows normally, there is a convexity forward in the cervical region from increased muscular power, as the head is held erect, the dorsal con-

[47] Lovett: Trans., Amer. Orthop. Assoc., vol. x, p. 22.

vexity backward lessens somewhat and as the thighs are extended and the child stands the pelvis tilts downward and forward producing the normal convexity forward in the lumbar region. Now should anything occur to lessen the power of the intrinsic spinal muscles or cause weakness, more or less deformity will occur, as the attitude departs from the normal. Various habitual attitudes and occupations tend to produce "round shoulders" or "round back," known as a "postural kyphosis," which is seen in children and adults alike, but it is more easily corrected in the former than the latter, before bony changes from functional transformations and osteosclerosis have occurred. Frequently when the dorsal kyphosis is much increased, lumbar lordosis becomes exaggerated compensatorily in maintaining the equilibrium and the child is not only stoop shouldered and narrow-chested, but sticks out the abdomen in an awkward unsightly manner. This is spoken of as a "hollow-roundback;" at times we see the manifestation of weakness chiefly, as a lordosis with swayback and prominent abdomen alone. The ætiology can be put down to faulty attitudes in sitting, reading and standing, poor respiration due to obstruction to chest expansion from adenoids, enlarged tonsils, bronchitis, heart

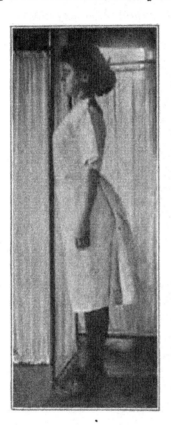

Fig. 77. Learning the Proper Standing Position.

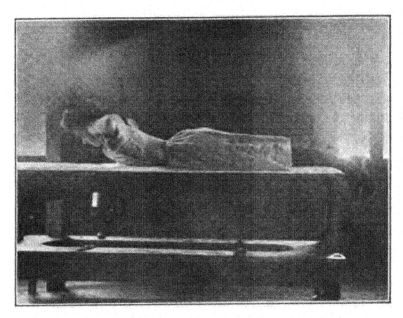

FIG. 78. STRENGTHENING THE ERECTOR SPINÆ, TRAPEZIUS AND RHOMBOIDS.

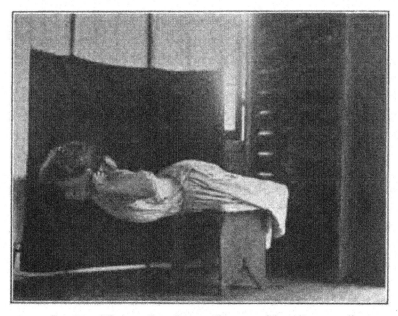

FIG. 79. "PRONE, LEG LYING, HOLDING, WING POSITION."

disease, clothing too tight across the thorax or dragging down unduly on the shoulders and sedentary habits, producing muscular weakness and atony.

Faulty attitudes will be mentioned more at length, in connection with the ætiology of lateral curvature of the spine, but suffice to say at this time the more common malpositions assumed by children in sitting is the tendency to lie down in chairs by sitting on the anterior edge, so that the middle and lower portions of the spine are unsupported; this of course tends to round back and stoop shoulders. (Figs. 75 and 76.) Another evil tendency is that seen at the school desk which is too low and leads to round shoulders, as the scholar stoops over or leans on it. Carrying the hands in the trousers pockets is another vicious habit in boys leading to contracture of the chest. Sleeping on the side, with legs drawn up and not on the back without a pillow, tends to stretch and weaken the posterior spinal muscles, besides interfering with the proper expansion of the lungs and development of the respiratory muscles. Slouching in standing and walking, standing on one foot and not bearing the weight equally on both, may increase the tendency to relaxation.

It is a common error for mothers of children with weak backs to feel that all of the clothing must depend from the shoulders, which already tend to stoop, instead of relieving them of any weight possible by making the hips do all they can to lessen this drag downwards. If shoulder straps are used to support garments they should be held by a cross strap to bring them as near the neck as possible, so as to have less leverage on the movable shoulder in producing malposition.[a] These common errors are mentioned so that they may be eliminated, as ætiological factors in producing or increasing the deformity.

[a] Goldthwait: Trans., Amer. Orthopædic Assoc

Treatment consists of a drill in a military attitude with head erect, chin in, chest out, stomach drawn in and feet pointing well forward. A convenient way to teach a child to assume this attitude is to have him stand with his toes about two inches from the edge of a door and have the

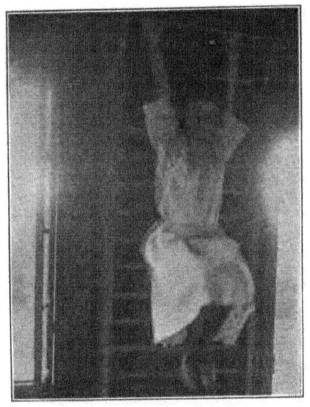

FIG. 80. "HOOK HANGING."

thorax touch it, but the nose and abdomen are to be held back from it. (Fig. 77.) While maintaining this attitude, the patient should daily or twice daily do various exercises and Swedish movements, which are most useful and essential to strengthen the unduly weak muscles in these conditions, such as,

(a) Free exercises in extending the arms in turn, upward, outward and downward rapidly and fully. Also backward as in swimming.

(b) Lying prone with the head and shoulders over the edge of a table, in the corrected position. (Fig. 78.)

(c) With the hands on the back of the neck, the elbows

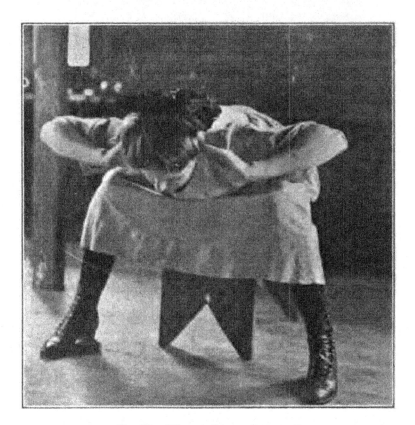

FIG. 81. "PRONE STRIDE SITTING."

held well back, with the front of the thighs supported on a box and the feet held, make the patient maintain the trunk in a horizontal position, thus increasing the tone of the superficial and deep groups of back muscles. (Fig. 79.)

(*d*) Hanging from a bar with the legs flexed on the thighs to 90° and the thighs flexed on the body a like amount, straightens the dorsal kyphosis and lumbar lordosis as well. (Fig. 80.)

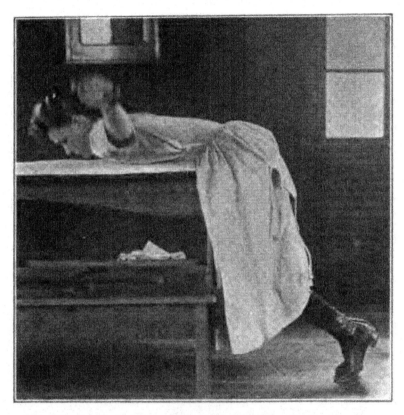

Fig. 82. An Exercise for Weak Trapezius and Rhomboids with Dumb-bells.

(*e*) Swinging the dumb-bells between the legs and upwards as high as possible strengthens all extensors.

(*f*) For lordosis due to flaccid abdominal muscles, lying on the back raising the legs vertically a number of times is an excellent exercise to increase abdominal muscular tone, when done from 45°.

(g) Teaching the child to take the position shown in Fig. 81, known as "prone stride sitting" with the arms in the wing position is very helpful in strengthening the spinal muscles and flattening the back.

(h) In Fig. 82 is shown an excellent means of strengthen-

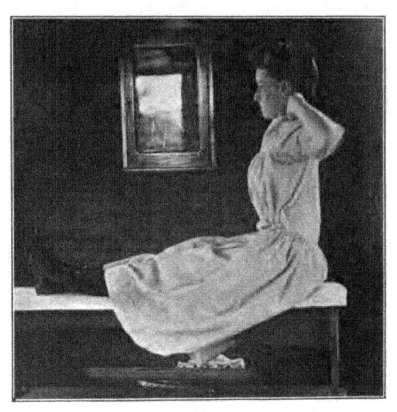

FIG. 83. AN EXERCISE FOR WEAK TRAPEZIUS, WEAK RHOMBOIDS AND LORDOSIS.

ing the posterior shoulder muscles by raising the arms up and down and increasing the effort by suitable dumb-bells held in the patient's hands which are to be raised and lowered in the plane of the shoulders.

(*i*)   "Long sitting, wing position" is another useful drill to use daily in overcoming tendencies to round shoulders and swayback.   (Fig. 83.)

(*j*)   In very many cases of kyphosis such contraction of the pectorals (major and minor) has occurred from prolonged faulty position, that it is essential to stretch them thoroughly before it is possible for the patient to assume

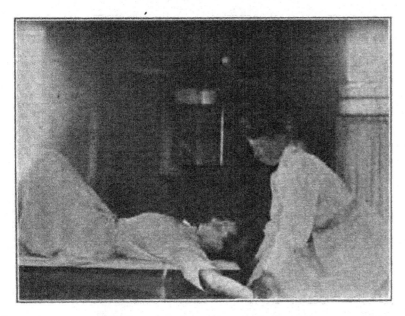

FIG. 84.   AN EXERCISE TO STRETCH CONTRACTED PECTORALS, GIVEN FORCIBLY BY GYMNAST WITH A PAD UNDER APEX OF KYPHOSIS.

anything like a proper position.   One method of doing this is shown in Fig. 84, where patient is in the "stretch grasp, hook lying" position and the gymnast forcibly carries the extended arms downward and backward.   The stretching can be facilitated by having a padded block between the shoulder blades.

Another method to accomplish this is to have the patient hang on the bar or "boom" with the hands as far apart as possible and for the gymnast to exert forcible forward pressure between the shoulder blades.

In some cases we find forcible hyperextension on the

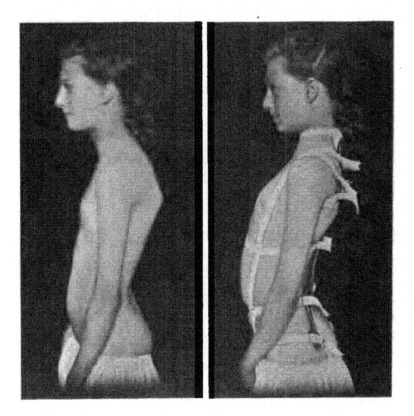

FIG. 85.   BEFORE AND DURING TREATMENT FOR KYPHO-LORDOSIS.

(Attention is directed to the improved nutrition of patient with better chest expansion and to the use of webbing straps on the brace instead of an "apron.")

kyphotone for twenty minutes or half an hour helpful in stretching daily these contracted muscles.

An exercise to correct forward thrusting of the head and neck, as seen in Figs. 85 and 86, is "reach, grasp standing, head extension with resistance." In this the patient faces the wall at arm's length with palms against the wall on a level with the shoulders and the head is extended backwards, while the gymnast resists. The chin should be held

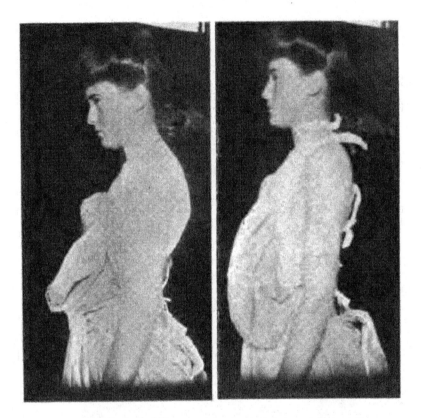

FIG. 86. CERVICO-DORSAL "ROUND BACK" BEFORE AND DURING TREATMENT, SHOWING EFFECT ON THE APPEARANCE OF THE BRACE.

against the throat when this is done. This exercise is to be repeated again and again.

In some cases that seem too weak to be able to hold erect, or in children who will not make a voluntary effort to maintain an improved position, a light steel back brace must be used in conjunction with the exercises, but it is better to do without it, if possible. It should be simply a light C. F. Taylor back brace, such as is used in Pott's

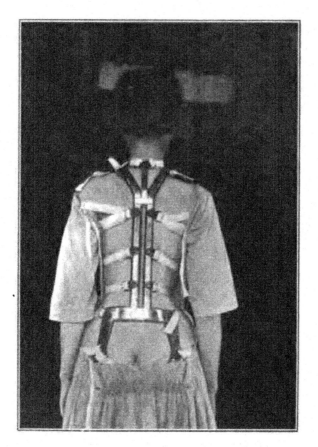

FIG. 87 THE MODIFIED C. F. TAYLOR BRACE FOR ROUND SHOULDERS AND FORWARD THRUSTING NECK.

Disease, with webbing straps instead of an apron, and with a throat strap if the neck is thrust forward. (Figs. 85, 86 and 87.)

CHAPTER VII.

NON-TUBERCULOUS DISEASES OF THE SPINE.—Continued.

LATERAL CURVATURE OF THE SPINE.

Definition. Lateral curvature is a deviation of a portion of or the entire spinal column to one or the other side or both sides of the vertical plane of the body, which usually causes more or less rotation of the vertebræ from which the ribs, transverse processes and muscles of one side may project backwards more than the other. One shoulder or one hip is commonly more prominent than the other.

Synonyms. Scoliosis and rotary lateral curvature.

Varieties. I. Congenital is seen; from 1. Fœtal rickets (rare). 2. Unequal development of the two sides of the thorax or inequality in the length of the legs or height of pelvic brim or "numerical variation" of the vertebræ.[a]

II. Acquired, being the commoner of the two and the one usually understood, from 1. Debility. 2. Faulty attitudes. 3. Empyema. 4. Paralysis. 5. Distortion of the pelvis as sequela of rickets. 6. Rachitic changes in the spine itself. 7. Distortion of the pelvis from asymmetrical muscular pull. 8. Physiological transformation to meet pathological function.

The occurrence is chiefly during the growing years. The age, when the cases are presented for treatment, is usually from the eighth to the fifteenth year.

Fifty per cent of the cases occur in the period from the first to the twelfth year approximately.

[a] Dwight, Rosenberg and Böhm. (*vide infra.*)

Forty per cent of the cases occur in the period from the twelfth to the fifteenth year.

Ten per cent of the cases occur in the period from the fifteenth year upwards.

Frequency. It occurs to a slight extent in a large number of individuals unrecognized; of deformities it forms from 20 to 30 per cent.

Sex. Four girls to every boy is about the proportion in which it is seen. Boys have nothing like the attention paid to their figures that girls do, hence they are less frequently brought to the surgeon's care for this trouble, unless the deformity is quite marked, and therefore statistics may be faulty on this point. Girls are more liable to form sedentary habits, taking less exercise and growing more rapidly than boys.

STAGES OF THIS AFFECTION.

There are three stages of lateral curvature.

I. *Initial stage.* This stage is not as a rule seen by the surgeon, as the deformity is not discovered by the parents until about the time of puberty. It occurs earlier, but is not recognized. Often the dressmaker will comment on the inequality of the two sides in waist or skirt or both. The slight elevation of one shoulder or prominence of one hip is first noted and the patient seems to bear more weight on one side habitually in sitting or standing than on the other. Inclination of the trunk to one side may be seen. Unequal muscular strength on the two sides is not the rule, although apparent from the child standing habitually on one leg. (Fig. 88.)

II. The stage of development is that in which the surgeon is usually consulted for the marked distortion, which has taken place as (1) a flexible or (2) fixed curvature.

A flexible curvature disappears on suspension or recumbency, as it is due to muscular or ligamentous relaxation, while a fixed curvature due to bony metamorphosis does not. A flexible curvature may be voluntarily corrected by the patient when taught to stand straight. A fixed curvature is sometimes called a structural curvature, implying permanent bony change. (Fig. 89.)

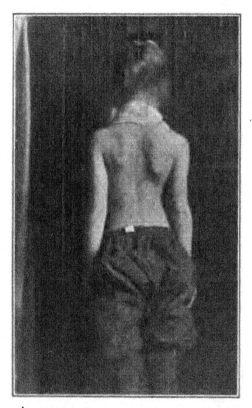

FIG. 88. A BEGINNING LEFT DORSO–LUMBAR "C" FLEXIBLE CURVATURE.

In the majority of cases the muscular system is poorly developed.

Nothing is complained of but the deformity, which varies greatly in the progress it has made. In growing girls we may find fatigue in standing or walking, perhaps neurasthenic pains in the back, legs or chest.

III. The stage of arrest cannot be sharply separated from the second stage, but it is usually considered as reached, when the time of osseous development is completed.

SYMPTOMS.

Symptoms are not the rule in this affection.

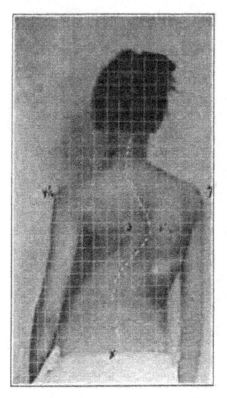

Fig. 89. A Right Dorsal and Left Lumbar "S" Fixed Curvature.

1. Pain may be present, but it is not proportionate to the deformity; if present, is usually in the lumbar region and thighs and worse from fatigue, as "backache."

Pain may be due to: (1) muscular or ligamentous strain. (2) Pressure from distorted ribs or change in the shape of the thorax with displacement of viscera, thoracic or abdominal (enteroptosis). (3) Neurasthenia and lowered vitality from lack of exercise. In severe disease in the debilitated, pain as a paræsthesia or hyperæsthesia, neuralgia, etc., may be complained of.

II. Interference with the functions of the stomach, liver and intestines in severe cases is rare. Gastroptosis with fermentative dyspepsia is at times a troublesome complication.

III. Dyspnœa may be present and is common in severe cases.

IV. Asthenia is seen in the worst types of the affection. In the worst form of this affection that came under the author's observation the patient could only lie down to sleep when a corrective jacket was worn, from interference with the heart's action, due to stenosis of the aorta, with mitral and tricuspid incompetency, following the curvature.

V. Limping is caused in severe cases by a tilting of the pelvis upward secondarily, making one leg shorter than the other, but this is extremely rare.

VI. Subcutaneous fat is markedly diminished often in severe cases, owing to general impairment of the respiratory and other bodily functions.

PHYSICAL SIGNS.

The physical signs on the other hand are marked.

I. The deformity is the lateral leaning or twisting of the spine. The deformity in mild cases may cause no signs in a casual examination save the prominence of the hip on one side and the elevation of the shoulder on the other, which causes a sensitiveness often unwarranted in a patient, as [the condition is not generally recognized. Compensatory curves may or may not be above or below the primary curve, or both, leading to "single," "total," "C" or double

"S"-shaped curves.   Prominence of the hip is due to rotation of the ribs forward on that side and the leaning of the whole trunk to the opposite side.   A simple "C" curvature may involve the entire dorsal and lumbar regions as a curvature to the right (or left) with rotation backward of the ribs on the same side, which is usually the right.

Primary cervical or high-dorsal curves are rare except with torticollis; when present there is a long compensatory curve, in the opposite direction below.   The head and face are held toward the concave side and the shoulder of the convex side is elevated and the opposite shoulder seems longer on the concave side.

Dorsal curvature is commonly convex to the right.   In these cases usually the right shoulder is raised, the right scapula is on a higher plane horizontally than the left, and is pulled further away from the spinal column.   The left shoulder is lowered and the scapula approaches nearer the median line.   The thorax below the left scapula is flattened or hollowed, while the right side of the back is rounded, from the rotation backwards of the ribs on the latter side and forwards on the former.

In the left dorsal curve the reverse takes place.

In front, in well-marked cases of right convex dorsal curvature, the left breast is more prominent than the right, owing to rotation of the ribs and falling of the shoulder.   The whole trunk may lean to the right, and the right arm swing free from the side and the left hang down against the pelvis. The contour of the back is asymmetrical, the right side is rounded with a hollow above the pelvis, while the left is flattened and sunken above and rounded in the lumbar region with a prominent hip on that side, i. e., "long waisted on the left side," as the patient expresses it.   These minor changes in the contour of the hips and shoulders, however, depend on the location of the spinal curvature; a low dorsal being very different from a high dorsal in its effect, for a low right dorsal may give a high left shoulder from a compensatory left cervico-dorsal curve.

Lumbar curvature gives a prominence of the hip (as a rule in double curvature) on the convex side of the dorsal curve. Similarly in a long lumbar curve simply, we may find the prominent hip on the concave side of the lumbar curve. But few cases are exactly similar in their physical appearance. The rotation backward of the transverse processes in the lumbar region occurs over the, or on the side of the, convexity, which is usually the left; in these cases, the umbilicus is to the right of the medial line. The contour of the back is, therefore, as in dorsal curvature, full or rounded over the convex side and flattened or hollowed over the concave side.

It is impossible to separate low dorsal and lumbar curvatures as the resulting deformity is the same, but the distortion of the more pronounced curve predominates.

A double curvature is one where two curves with their resulting distortions are equal. In it the leaning to one side is not as marked as in a simple dorsal curvature.

Rotation or Torsion. In order for a curvature in the spine to occur laterally, a certain amount of rotation or torsion of the vertebræ on themselves *must take place.* The amount of this is the guide to the severity of the case as it results in a twisting of the ribs (through their attachments to the transverse processes), and as the ribs rotate backward they lift the scapula of that side causing elevation of a shoulder and vice versa; lower down this vertebral twist causes prominence of the transverse processes with the lumbar muscles, but of course not of the same degree as that seen in the region of the ribs. Torsion may be the first sign noted even before any deviation of the line in the spinous processes is seen, as they may rotate around a line joining the spinous processes as an axis.

SEAT OF THE DISTORTION.

Authorities differ at to whether lumbar or dorsal scoliosis is the more common, but the "prominent shoulder
blade" (in dorsal curvature) is usually responsible for the
parent seeking advice of the surgeon, hence our statistics
would indicate dorsal as the most frequent.

Approximately three-fourths of the cases seen have one
chief curve; over half of these cases are in the dorsal region
and are convex to the right; about one-third of the cases have
a double curve, and two-thirds of these cases have the
upper curve to the right and the lower curve to the left.

Left lateral dorsal curve is commoner in flexible young
children.

VARIETIES DEPENDING ON THE CAUSE.

1. Caries in the early stages of Pott's Disease as pointed
out under that subject may lead to scoliosis from breaking
down of one side of one or more vertebral bodies.

2. Caries with irregular ossification in old neglected healed
cases of Pott's Disease may produce scoliosis as may

3. Spondylolisthesis with dislocation or fracture of the
vertebræ.

4. Torticollis and sacro-iliac disease may lead to a postural form of the affection.

5. Rickets may lead to a scoliotic curve, although it is
not as common as the rachitic kyphosis. When present
is usually to the left. About 10 per cent of the rachitic
have it. Usually in more than half of the cases it appears
in the first six months of life, but may be overlooked and
discovered when the child begins to grow more rapidly from
the eighth to the fifteenth year

It may be present without any other signs of rickets and
is of equal frequency in boys and girls. Lateral curvature
may lead to an antero-posterior curve from the unequal dis-

tribution of weight with marked unilateral kyphosis above and lordosis below.

6. The static form occurs from congenital, traumatic or pathological inequality in the length of the legs or the shape of the pelvis in about one-fourth of the cases seen, and of these three-fourths have the left leg the shorter. This

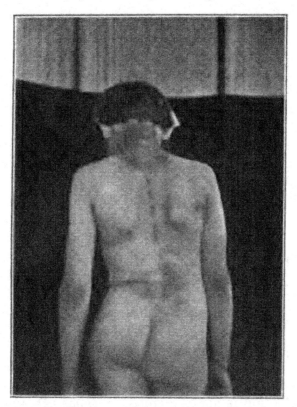

FIG. 90. A RIGHT LUMBAR CURVATURE DUE TO A SHORT RIGHT LEG.

shortening may be due to infantile paralysis, knock-knee, hip disease, flat-foot, habitual unequal muscular pull, etc. (Fig. 90.)

Simply habitual faulty attitude in standing on one leg or leaning to one side is supposed to cause a variety of scoliosis.

Lowered vitality with organic changes in the tissues associated with faulty attitude may cause backache and pain in the onset of lateral curvature.

7. Unilateral paralysis of the back muscles due to infantile paralysis, or progressive muscular atrophy, etc., may cause the patient to assume a position which will cause the least possible strain to the muscles and result in scoliosis, with the convexity *towards the paralyzed or non-resisting side,* from contraction of those in which the tone is still good on the other side. Friedrich's ataxia is also frequently accompanied by scoliosis as a symptom as well as by club-foot.

8. Empyema may cause connective tissue contraction, loss of expansibility of the lung on the diseased side and increased expansion of the other, which pulls the vertebræ *over to the healthy side.* Loss of a rib or ribs after Estländer's operation may cause scoliosis. It is not a true scoliosis, however, but may lead to a true lateral curvature with rotation from the altered position and function of the spine (functional pathogenesis of deformity).

In all cases the ribs are lowered on the diseased side.

9. Pneumonia and phthisis are rarely a cause. An heredity of lateral curvature with an heredity of phthisis may lead to a rapid deformity without phthisis. An heredity predisposition to scoliosis or some form of spinal curvature is found in from one-fourth to one-half of the cases.

10. Sarcoma of the lungs and ribs has been reported as an ætiological factor.

11. Occupation is not as common a cause as would seem, as the laborious occupations are entered upon after ossific hardening has occurred. Examples of it, however, are found in *school children* (hence the play on the word, "schooliosis"), clerks, blacksmiths, hod and basket carriers. Infants may develop scoliosis from one sided nursing by hemiplegic mothers, according to Bradford and Lovett.

The curvature of course depends on the character of the occupation.

12. Unequal eyesight may lead to it from an habitual vicious attitude, chiefly seen as a torticollis or cervical curvature with compensatory curves below. This defective carriage of the head has been called attention to by George Gould and Augustus Wilson, and glasses should not be fitted by oculists except with the head held straight.

13. Sciatica may cause a lumbar curve.

14. A "physiological" lateral curve is sometimes seen in right-handed people and some authorities hold it is from the weight of the heart. Left-handed people may have a high shoulder.

THEORIES AS TO THE ÆTIOLOGY OF SCOLIOSIS.

1. *Unequal Muscular Action.* By some this is considered the same mechanical condition that is seen in torticollis, but this is questioned by others, as there is no spasm on the concave side of the scoliosis. Many think a weakened condition of the muscles on the convex side is the cause, but in opposition to this is the fact that lateral curvature is seen in the strongly muscled occasionally. In delicate people habits of attitude may weaken certain muscles by overstretching and this is also seen in the paralytics. However, muscular weakness may be considered a predisposing influence if not an actual cause of the deformity. The muscles, primarily involved, it is supposed by some are the deep group of the erector spinæ muscles, *i. e.*, those attached from segment to segment ("intrinsic spinal muscles," Shaffer).

Mackenzie[a] first called attention to the male type of pelvis on one side and the female type on the other in scoliosis with unequal muscular pull.

[a] Trans. Amer. Orthopædic Assoc., vol. vii, p. 343, 1894.

Riely[46] then pointed out that there is a congenital or acquired rachitic distortion in the crests of the ilia in a large number of cases, so that there is a greater pull on the ribs by the abdominal muscles on one side than on the other and this causes not only the scoliosis but the rotation. The pelvis on one side is of the male type and on the other of the female type. He has also stated that the ilium on one side is tilted not only downward and outward, but downward and forward more than its mate, so that measurements taken from the anterior iliac spines to determine the length of the legs give erroneous results.

It is an error he claims to attribute scoliosis to defective action of the deep groups of dorsal muscles with their insufficient leverage on the transverse and spinous processes and that the superficial groups are chiefly concerned with shoulder and arm movements.

He feels that the *abdominal muscles pulling on those long levers, the ribs, asymmetrically* from a distorted pelvis, may not only effect a torsion of the vertebræ, but a lateral deviation as well.

Now whether, as Riely seems to think, an asymmetrical pelvis is the primary cause or whether an habitual faulty attitude, as the author feels[47] distorts the pelvis and throws the abdominal muscles into one sided action and the spine out of equilibrium, one cannot say. We do know and *have seen pathologically in cases of unilateral coxa vara, and congenital hip dislocation, how the pelves are distorted by abnormal and asymmetrical muscular pull,* and we must bear in mind that the ossification between the ilium, ischium and pubes by means of the Y-cartilage does not begin until the thirteenth or fourteenth year and is not complete until the twenty-fifth year. The ilium could be pulled in or out as

[46]Journal Amer. Med. Assoc., April 2, 1904.
[47]American Jour. Orthopædic Surgery, Jan., 1905.

the case may be by an habitual tension of the muscles in
one direction.   The harm is done usually before the thirteenth or fourteenth [year, as the cases are presented for
treatment usually at or before that time.

2. Unilateral hypertrophy and atrophy of vertebræ.
(Volkmann-Hueter.)

Asymmetrical osseous development, as is seen in genu-
valgum, or ligamentous changes with early ossification of
one side some hold is the cause and not the effect of the
vicious attitude.   This, however, cannot be proven clinically
or pathologically.

3. Functional pathogenesis of deformity.   Wolff proves
"functional use" in the changed or deformed position is
responsible for the pathogenesis of the bone deformity and
osteosclerosis results on the concave side and osteoporosis
on the convex and this is probably the correct view of the
resulting changes in the vertebræ seen in the fixed curvatures.

Superincumbent weight, pressing on a faulty position of
the vertebral column, is the theory that receives the widest
acceptance, causing perverted or what we may call pathological function, which leads to bone change.   This begins
to act in childhood as a vicious attitude with at first a
flexible spine, which later becomes fixed from the adaptive
shortening of muscles and ligaments, and results in changes
in the shapes of the bony structures from the pressure of
superincumbent weight, as claimed by those who do not hold
Wolff's views, and physiological bone transformation to meet
pathological static demands by those who agree with him.

4. Max Böhm,[a] in a very interesting anatomical, rönt-
genological and clinical research, has shown conclusively that
a large number of cases of so-called "habitual scoliosis,"
or those supposed to be due to vicious habit, can be traced

[a]Boston Med. and Surg. Jour., vol. cliv, no. 4, p. 99, and clv, no. 21, p. 598.

back to defective asymmetrical embryological development of the vertebræ or ribs of the atavistic (or lower species) type or the epigonistic (or higher species) type.

Dwight[*] called attention to the "numerical variations" in the human spine by which is meant "variations in a cranial direction," where the ribs begin to be attached to the seventh cervical vertebra instead of the first dorsal or the ilium is attached to the fifth lumbar vertebra instead of to the first sacral, or where the first dorsal articular processes resemble the cervical processes or the first lumbar the dorsal or first sacral the lumbar, etc., and "variations in the caudal direction" would be the reverse of these in a downward direction.

Böhm having the advantage of the study of Dwight's anatomical collection of 54 spines, that showed these variations, together with X-ray pictures of a series of cases of scoliosis showing these variations also *asymmetrically*, put two and two together very ingeniously and states that the cause of scoliosis in very many of these cases which we see in the developing second decade of life date back to an embryological defect. Thus he showed, for example, in X-rays a partial development of a sixth lumbar or transitional sacral vertebra on the right side with a higher attachment of the ilium on the left side, and consequent left lumbar scoliosis; an imperfect articulation between dorsal and lumbar vertebra on *one* side and consequent sag or curvature of that side; unilateral cervical or lumbar ribs with consequent lateral concavity to the opposite side, etc. It is quite possible as he points out to imagine and recognize one or several of these variations in one individual producing compensatory or structural S-curves.

One can but praise the logic of Böhm's reasoning and the value of his work and actual demonstrations; at the same

[*] Memoirs of the Boston Society of Natural History, vol. v, 1901.

time we must bear in mind, certainly in the less severe structural cases, that physiological bone transformation can take place as the result of persistent faulty positions, so that we may get from this cause also a distinct "variation" from the characteristic type of a certain vertebral group. This may be said especially with regard to the articular processes and bodies. Further in viewing the radiographs *unless this is done stereoscopically*, one may fall into errors in judging the shape of rotated vertebræ or whether a rib is seen on the flat or edgewise. The rotation which is always present in these cases causes distortions in *flat* outlines which are confusing. Böhm suggests that instead of using the term "habitual" lateral curvature we should speak of these cases as "delayed congenital scoliosis" or "scoliosis congenitalis tarda." His observation is most important and adds one more ætiological factor to our list.

5. *Age.* Childhood is the time when from whatever cause these osseous changes and rapid growth occur and predisposes to the production of this condition.

CAUSES IN GENERAL.

Causes may be stated as: 1. Predisposing from debility, rickets, defective development, childhood, etc. 2. Exciting which disturb the equilibrium, such as vicious attitudes, paralysis, empyema, etc.

PATHOLOGY.

Pathological changes do not result from disease but from pressure and improper functional use of bones that yield. In bad cases all the bones of the trunk may be involved, including the pelvis, primarily or secondarily, but the change is seen most markedly in the bodies, articular and transverse processes of the vertebræ and the ribs. The changes vary according to the amount of the curvature and

rotation.   Muscles and ligaments are altered only in tonic-
ity and length, for degenerative changes occur only later
in the severest cases.   The writer found even in the normal
spines of a large number examined and measured for Dr.
Bradford at the Warren Museum of the Harvard Medical
School, that the two sides of the individual vertebræ were
not symmetrical.   In scoliosis, after the flexible stage has
passed into the fixed stage, this asymmetry becomes greatly
exaggerated.   In the fixed stage, it is found on the concave
side of the curve, that the bodies of the vertebræ are less
thick than on the convex.   They, therefore have received

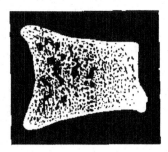

FIG. 91.   A CROSS SECTION OF A "SCOLIOTIC WEDGE," SHOWING OSTEOSCLEROSIS
ON CONVEX SIDE AND OSTEOPOROSIS ON CONCAVE.

the name of the "scoliotic wedges."   This change in shape
is brought about by physiological processes, as pointed out
by Wolff, to meet pathological static demands of pressure,
torsion and shearing strain and results not in an atrophy
of the concave side, as formerly taught under the Volkmann-
Heuter hypothesis, but of a condensation or osteosclerosis
of the trabeculæ to stand increased weight bearing and a
trabecular resorption or osteoporosis on the convex side on
which less strain is put.   (Fig. 91.)   Wolff has clearly shown
that the external contour and internal architecture in bones
are mutually dependent on the function demanded.

The intervertebral cartilages undergo similar wedge shape changes and one can well understand that any column made up of quadrilaterally shaped bodies (on section), upon being made into an arc, would necessitate the side of each body on the concave side of the curve becoming narrower than the side on the convex.

The changes in the shapes of the spinous, articular and transverse processes are explained chiefly by the torsion which invariably takes place in scoliosis. This is brought about by the resistance experienced by bones from ligamentous and muscular attachment, thus if the vertebral body is rotated to the right, the muscular and ligamentous attach-

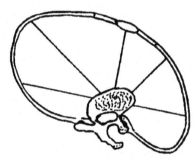

FIG. 92.   CROSS SECTION OF THORAX IN REGION OF RIGHT DORSAL SCOLIOSIS.
(Hoffa.)

ments resist a coincident rotation of the spinous process to the left and hence the spinous process gradually yields partially and becomes curved somewhat to the right, so that its tip is no longer directly in an imaginary line drawn from the center of the posterior edge of the vertebral body, but to the right of it.   (Fig. 92.)

Similarly, in the dorsal region, the ribs being attached by strong ligaments to the transverse processes can permit of little movement of the latter in which they do not participate, so that when any rotation backward of a transverse process occurs its rib is carried backward also and the costal angle becomes bent more acutely, while the corresponding rib is carried forward and its angle flattened out or rendered more obtuse. The ribs are not only rotated forward or backward and changed in shape, but they are directed upward or downward, as the case may be, and are further apart on the convex side than on the concave. (Fig. 93.)

Pari passu with these changes the tip of the sternum may be deflected toward the side of the dorsal convexity.

Even in severe cases but little change occurs in the clavicles, although the external half of a right clavicle may be more curved than normal in severe right dorsal scoliosis. The scapula on the side of the dorsal convexity is unduly elevated by the backward protruding ribs and removed outward from the median line, while the other scapula having its costal support withdrawn sinks downward and its inferior angle approaches abnormally near the spinal column; the scapula over the convexity is more concave and that over the concavity is more flattened than normal.

The thorax is therefore necessarily much distorted over the convex curve in the back where the ribs project or bulge abnormally backward, while on the opposite side, it is flattened or hollowed. (Fig. 94.) In front the reverse occurs and in larger girls the mamma corresponding with the concave side of the dorsal curve is the more prominent. The umbilicus may be deflected from the median line. When rotation occurs in the lumbar region where no ribs are attached, the deformity is not so marked, but some of the lumbar muscles project on the convex side and are depressed on the other, as has been stated under physical signs. Thus the contour of that region is slightly altered comparatively with the dorsal region and the trouble is evident chiefly in an increased furrow above one hip making it more prominent and the individual seeming "longer waisted" on the convex side. (Fig. 89.)

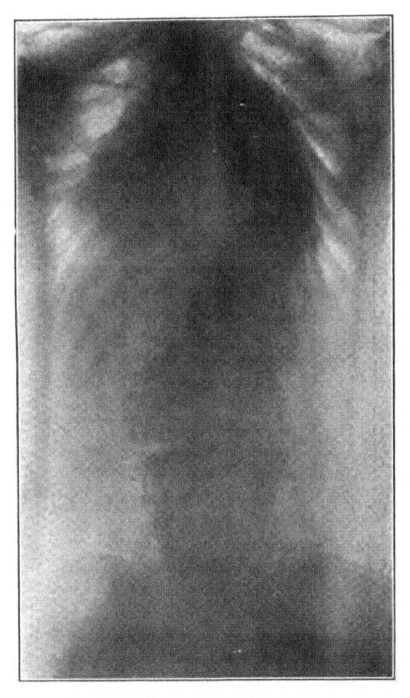

Fig. 93.   X-ray of an S-Shaped Scoliosis.

Note the greater separation of ribs on the right, wedge-shaped bodies and intervertebral cartilages; also a wedge-shaped *6th* lumbar vertebra.

In the severest fixed cases a formative osteitis may anky-
lose the articular processes of the vertebræ together.   The
capacity of that side of the thorax into which the convexity
projects is lessened as the bodies of the vertebræ encroach
more and more upon it and the ribs in front are flattened
and their angles decreased behind.   On the other hand the
diagonal diameter of the thorax from the ribs of the convex
side forward is greater than normal and that of the other

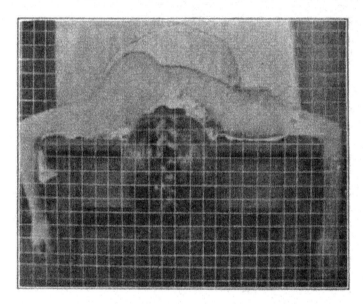

FIG. 94.   CASE SHOWN IN FIG. 88 SIGHTED DOWN THE BACK, SHOWING MARKED
ROTATION BACKWARD OF RIBS ON THE RIGHT SIDE.

side less.   (Fig. 92.)   In very severe cases, the ribs on the
concave side may sink into the pelvis and change the shape
of its bones; this is especially true in cases where there is
marked inclination of the trunk to the opposite side.

The muscles and ligaments as stated are only found
changed in the severest cases; degeneration of the former
occurs first on the concave side with adaptive shortening
of the ligaments.   (Phelps.)

Prominence of the dorsal and lumbar muscles in scoliosis has been mistaken for abscess and incised or explored with an aspirator. Neither compression of the spinal nerves (owing to the large size of the foremina) nor are changes in the spinal cord liable to occur in scoliosis. Berg was unable to detect any reaction of degeneration in the nerves supplying the "extrinsic" spinal muscles, *i. e.*, the superficial group of back muscles.

The thoracic viscera are more often displaced than the abdominal and the capacity of the chest, as was shown above, of one side may be smaller than the other, but no statistics of phthisis exist as a consequence. The liver may be displaced, the spleen compressed and the greater curvature of the stomach may be near or below the umbilicus in the cases of enteroptosis complicating this condition.

Unlike reptiles and fish as types possessing the most marked power of lateral bending of the vertebral column, the human spine, except in infancy, and to a still less degree in old age, has but little without a coincident twisting or rotation owing to the shape of its integral parts. The ligamentous attachments between the parallel transverse and spinous processes also limit lateral bending.

Motions, however, in flexion and extension can be executed easily normally and in certain regions rotation readily occurs.

At the occipito-atlantoidal articulation we have all three motions, namely, flexion, lateral bending and to a lesser degree rotation.

At the atlanto-axoid articulation we have chiefly rotation.

The remaining cervical vertebræ, on account of the concavo-convex superposition of the bodies, which are longer transversely than antero-posteriorly and the transversely articulating articular processes, permit motions chiefly in flexion and extension and these very conditions together with the horizontal overlapping transverse and spinous processes with their anchoring ligaments and muscles check motions in rotation and lateral bending.

When we examine the dorsal vertebræ we find on the other hand spherical or heart-shaped bodies (with the apex anterior), obliquely articulating articular processes and oblique or vertical overlapping spinous processes so that rotation and lateral oblique bending can more easily take place, and flexion is more limited than elsewhere in the spine.

In the lumbar region the shape and relation of the vertebræ and the mechanical function are quite similar to the lower cervical region, namely, that flexion and extension are more natural than rotation or lateral bending, although the last two are more commonly seen and to a greater degree in the lumbar than the cervical region.

Thus it is easy to understand why the rotation is so much more marked in the dorsal region than in the others.

As in every kyphosis we have a compensatory lordosis, so in a backward rotation in the upper part of the spine to the right, by the law of compensation we must have a backward rotation to the *left* below and vice versa.

DIAGNOSIS.

In slight cases, diagnosis is only made on careful examination. In severe cases it is evident at a glance. To systematically examine a case, the back should be bared by stripping the patient to the trochanters. Mark the tips of the spinous processes, the inferior angles of the scapulæ, crests of the ilia and anterior and posterior superior iliac spines with a skin pencil. Attach by means of a surgeon's plaster, a plumb line to the seventh cervical vertebra. Then one can measure any deviation, if present, of the spinous processes and any difference in the distance of the two inferior scapular angles from the vertical line and the height one is above the other.   Note any projection or difference in contour of the two sides of the thorax and lumbar region as seen from behind.   Also any elevation of a shoulder or prominence of a hip or mamma and deviation of xiphoid cartilage or umbilicus from the median line of the body.   Then note any asymmetry that exists when the patient is viewed from above, or when stooping over is viewed from below.   Examine the amount of flexibility of the spine by holding the pelvis when the patient sits or stands, and then bends laterally as far as possible.   Also one may test the flexibility of the lumbar spines by placing as many one-half inch blocks as possible under each foot without flexing the knees, but with both legs straight.   This is to be done first on one side then on the other.

The possible rotation flexibility of a spine is to be tested by having patient sit on a revolving stool and turn while the shoulders are fixed.   (Bradford and Lovett.)   "Fixed" rotation is determined by making the patient lie recumbent or by suspension, when if "flexible" and not "fixed," the asymmetry of the ribs, etc., and in the contour of the back will disappear.   Tests of strength of back, arms, shoulders, sides, etc., can be made by spring balance dynamometers, which with weight and height records can be compared with the tables of the average for that age.   (Bowditch's.) The length of the legs should be measured not only from the anterior superior spines of the ilia to the internal malleoli but from the major trochanters to the external malleoli and also from the highest point of the crest of the ilia to the external malleoli.   Flat foot on either side is also to be noted and taken into consideration.   The inclination of the pelvis on each side should also be determined by a suitable balance or level between the anterior and posterior iliac spines, such as the leveling trapezium of Schulthess.

RECORDS OF CASES.

Records can be kept by measuring the distance of the tips of the spinous processes, inferior scapular angles and points of greatest prominence from the plumb line (*vide supra*) and plotting on plotting paper.

The most convenient method is perhaps by means of photographs taken through a frame upon which at vertical and horizontal intervals of an inch cord or wire is stretched and the measurements can then be seen at once on the photographs in inches and any change would be apparent in the next photograph, if improvement or the reverse had resulted from treatment. (Figs. 88, 89 and 94.) The same light and shadows are to be used in subsequent photographs to avoid error and the position is to be the same especially with regard to the frame. Thus an exact record of each case can be kept from time to time. In the absence of photographs outline sketches made at stated intervals are of some value and the tracing apparatus of Schulthess is the most accurate of all.

The author would suggest the following method to determine the angle of rotation in scoliosis; the patient is made to lie prone on the examining table, the face turned to the left in right dorsal scoliosis and to the right in left dorsal curvature, with the arms at the side, palms of the hands down and the elbows as close to the body as possible.

A yard stick is placed across the spine at the point of greatest rotation with its center at the spinous process of that region, the vertical distance from the two extremities of this stick to the examining table or floor is then measured by a graduated rectangular triangle, such as one may obtain at a store where drawing instruments are sold.

Now in a symmetrical back these two extremities would be equidistant from the table or floor. The difference between the two, in distance from the table, in a rotated

NON-TUBERCULOUS DISEASES OF THE SPINE.

spine, would give the side of a rectangular triangle opposite
the angle to be determined, if we imagine a plane parallel
to the normal back plane or to the table as one side of the
triangle.

The normal plane of the back may be easily determined
in a rotated spine as it is the same distance below the upper
extremity of the yard stick that it is above the lower extremity of it. Suppose a beam to be perfectly balanced at its
center, each end would be equidistant from the ground;
this we may call the normal plane of the back. Now suppose this beam is rocked on its central point of balance,
which occurs in a, rotated spine, one will be as much above
the normal plane as the other is below it, and the diagonal
angles opposite made by the intersection of the rocked beam
with the normal plane will be equal. As the normal plane
is parallel with the ground, any angle formed with it, or
any parallel plane, will be the same as that formed with the
ground. Now this can readily be applied to the rotated
scoliotic spine in a prone position, for when any angle is made
by the rotated spine with the normal spinal plane the same
angle is made with the examining table or any plane parallel
to it, as is well known from geometry ("alternate interior
angles are equal").

Now to apply the yardstick method to the rotated spine:

In Fig. 96 CD represents the yardstick or plane of the
rotated spine with its center at B the spinous process and ET
the examining table or floor. Suppose CE is a longer vertical distance than DT (as determined by the graduated
rectangle triangle).

Now by subtracting DT from CE leaving CA and projecting an imaginary plane from A to D the line AD is parallel
to ET naturally, as it has been drawn through two points
equidistant from ET; further, CAD is a right angle, as CET
was and the distance CA is the side of a right angled tri-

angle opposite the angle of rotation to be determined, or the identical angle the plane of the rotated spine would make with the examining table or a prolongation of its surface.

Now if CE should equal DT, CD would be parallel to the examining table, coincide with NP and no angle would be made naturally and CD here would equal the normal plane of the normal back.

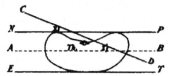

FIG. 95.   NORMAL PLANE OF THE BACK.

TH = normal thorax.
NP = normal plane of the back.
ET = examining table or ground.
AB = any plane parallel to NP and ET.
CD = any intersecting plane with NP and AB.
 X = X' or any corresponding angle made with ET.

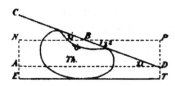

FIG. 96.   ANGLE OF ROTATION IN SCOLIOSIS.

Vertical distance CN = PD, as CB = BD.
$CE - DT$ = CA one side of a rectangular triangle.
Now CA is the side opposite the angle (X) of rotation sought.
$X = X' = X^2 = X^3$.

If on the other hand CE should be 36 inches longer than DT, we would have the yardstick vertical to the examining table and the angle of rotation of the spine would be 90 degrees.   From these two extremes it is easy to construct a working table.

If the distance in inches between CE and DT is	0	2	4	6	8	10	12	14	16	18	20	22	24	26	28	30	32	34	36
The angle in degrees is	0	5	10	15	20	25	30	35	40	45	50	55	60	65	70	75	80	85	90

Now in order to facilitate the working of this method the author has graduated the sides of the rectangular triangle in inches and had the above table put upon its hypothenuse.

Of course we all bear in mind the great difficulty of obtaining exact records of the rotation in scoliosis from the natural tendency for the body to assume dissimilar postures on different occasions when records are desired, but whether we use the ancient lead tape for tracings, or the weight bar and plumb of Bradford; or complicated machines such as that of Demeny or Schulthess, we will encounter this same source of error. The above method is not claimed as a perfect one and free of error, but its simplicity of application and the cheapness of the necessary instruments recommend it. Further, from the fact that the patient is to be prone, with the face always turned to one definite side, the palms of the hands down in contact with the examining table the elbows as close to the sides as possible and the lightness of the yardstick, the element of error at the varying periods of examination is minimized.

DIFFERENTIAL DIAGNOSIS.

From Pott's Disease, Lateral Curvature is distinguished by the absence, as a rule, of any acute antero-posterior angle, muscular spasm, pain, fixation of the spine (in early cases) and by the presence of rotation. When there is lateral deviation in Pott's Disease there is little rotation as a rule and a diagnosis of Pott's Disease has usually been made previously from the night-cries, attitude, pain, etc., even if a "knuckle" is not present. One practically never sees true scoliosis without rotation.

PROGNOSIS.

I. The prognosis without treatment, as to self-limitation or increase of the deformity, depends on:

1. The general health of the patient.

2. The severity and fixedness of the curve and the amount of rotation.

3. Rapidity of growth and an hereditary tendency to height are unfavorable.

4. The time of second dentition is especially unfavorable for the arrest of this condition. (A child grows more from the middle of July to the middle of November than at any other time of the year.)

5. Rickets or phthisis are unfavorable.

Spontaneous disappearance of the deformity in a growing child is most rare. Predictions of the rapidity of the increase of a deformity or the permanency of the arrest of the distortion should be most guarded. It is more common to see an increase in the growing years but it is also seen occasionally in slowly developing adults.

II. Prognosis with efficient treatment.

1. If the general health is good and even if the curve is very marked but flexible, it may become corrected. 2. The more rotation of course the more difficult the cure or marked improvement. 3. The position of the curve influences the efficiency of treatment. Dorsal curvature is the most difficult to treat. Lateral curvature in Pott's Disease in the earlier stages is easily corrected by suitable treatment of the primary disease (*vide supra*). In late Pott's Disease, where ossific changes and ankylosis have occurred, no treatment is available of course. In general it may be stated that with efficient treatment the increase in the fixed curvature may be checked and in the majority of cases there is marked improvement. In the severest and neglected cases the great aim should be to keep them from getting any worse and hold the deformity, at least.

TREATMENT.

Under the treatment of scoliosis, preventive measures will be considered first and then the treatment of developed cases.

PREVENTIVE MEASURES.

As faulty attitude plays such an important part in the development of scoliosis by destroying the equilibrium of the body and throwing a constant strain and stretch on one set of muscles thereby weakening it, while its fellow on the opposite side of the body is unduly relaxed, thereby undergoing adaptive shortening, attention to positions, habits of attitude and the like in growing children seems of the first importance, more especially where they are delicate or rapidly developing. These points may be noticed in the following ways:

1. *In Standing.* Habitual attitudes of throwing all the weight on one leg and not assuming the "attitude of rest" when the two legs are fully extended and bear the weight of the body equally, may be considered faulty and to be avoided. Proper balancing of the body should be taught, with head erect, chin in, shoulders back, chest thrown forward, hips back, feet adducted and legs sufficiently separated to afford an easy, comfortable equilibrium. This is the "attitude of rest." Weak children can be much helped in attaining this, by out-of-door exercises, gymnastics or Swedish movements, or home exercises under skilled supervision. Military schools will help in the case of boys. The keynote to all the exercises, however, should be to keep a correct balance, approaching the attitude of rest as nearly as possible, from which all standing exercises should be taken. In cases that stand with the weight thrown on one side from short leg, muscular weakness, a bad knee or ankle or flat foot suitable measures should be taken to correct these troubles by having the shoe sole thickened the desired

amount. When prolonged standing is necessary, as in church, school, etc., a weak child will find relief in advancing one foot *forward* or *backward* and still keep the spine erect. It is the placing of one foot *far to one side* and resting the weight entirely and habitually on the other leg that destroys the equilibrium. Cases have also come under the author's care with very severe right dorsal scoliosis from prolonged practicing on the violin, in those who had a predisposition to spinal weakness. The violin masters required these pupils to be able to see their left elbows under the body of the violin, thus throwing the dorsal and lumbar spine to the right of the median line. Folding the arms over the chest contracts it and is a bad habit as is, in boys, the habit of thrusting the hands into the trousers' pockets.

2. *In Walking.* The carriage should be symmetrical on the two sides and the head and trunk held as in standing, save the body may be flexed forward at the hips. The hands should not be carried in the pockets nor should one hand be used for carrying weights more than the other. Children come under observation who develop the habit of carrying one shoulder higher than the other from taking under one arm a large pile of school-books or bundles.

3. *Sitting.* Many faulty attitudes assumed by school children and children at home as well, may be considered as the cause of some of the cases of lateral curvature. These attitudes are more often than not the result of improper chairs and seats, or in other words, those that *do not fit and support the child.* A chair or school desk-seat should have a back with an inclination backward of 100 to 110 degrees with the seat. The seat proper should be as wide, generally speaking, as the child's thighs, including the buttocks, are long, from the flexed knee. There should be an inclined foot support for the fully extended legs either on the floor or attached to the chair. But perhaps most important of all, every chair

should have on the back as part of it, or attachable, a pad that fits exactly and supports well the lumbar region.[50] Piano and desk-stools should have backs that fit well into the lower dorsal and lumbar regions. A reclining chair should fit into the physiological curves of the spine and have a forward convexity under the occiput to fit into the cervical region as well as at the lumbar concavity. Reading and writing naturally come under this heading, and the position of the desk or table is important and its height should be proportioned to the person sitting. The distance from the top of the seat to the top of the table should be one-eighth the height of a girl and one-seventh that of a boy or two inches plus the distance from the olecranon of the semi-flexed forearm to the seat. The edge of the desk should be just over the edge of the seat. The inclination of the top of the desk should be a slope of two inches in a breadth of twelve.[51] Many different and faulty attitudes and twistings of the body are assumed in writing. Bradford and Lovett say: "The proper attitude during writing is with the transverse axis of the trunk parallel with the edge of the writing table. The forearms should rest for at least two-thirds of their length upon the table. The trunk should be held erect, the legs should be straight before the trunk and the feet should rest upon a sloping cricket, to support and steady the legs." (Figs. 75, 76, 97 and 98.)

4. *In Sleeping.* Statistics go to show that the most common attitude in sleep is faulty, *i. e.*, on one or the other side, although the dorsal decubitus is more common than upon either single side. A child should not be allowed to assume a twisted or contracted position and should be taught perferaby to sleep on its back, as freer chest expansion is thereby obtained from the dorsal attachment of the

---

[50] Staffel: Centralblatt f. orthop. Chir., May 1, 1885.
[51] Staffel: *Ibid.*

ribs to the spine.   In threatening cases, Bradford bed frames
may be used to ensure a proper position.   In a developed
case, the patient should sleep on the side of the greatest
concavity or the back.   A firm bed and no pillow should be
the rule.

5. *Corsets.*   Hutchinson[52] has shown that corsets weaken
the muscles of the trunk and are to be avoided in developing

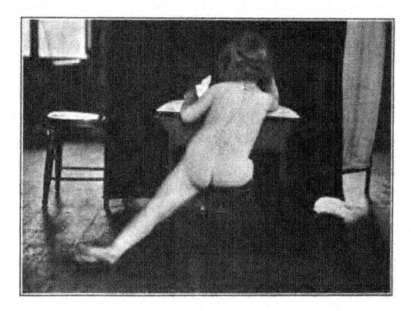

FIG. 97.   COMMON FAULTY ATTITUDE IN CHILDREN WHICH PRODUCES RIGHT DORSAL
AND LEFT LUMBAR CURVATURE IN SITTING.

girls.   The injury from corsets may be made less by having
elastic lacings and the waist without steels or supported by
light bones only.   Corsets are never the shape of the human
thorax and the prevailing mode of bloused waists render
their use entirely superfluous in the majority of cases.   The
less tone a girl has the more relaxed and flabby she is, the
more reason there should be for her not wearing corsets and

[52] Med. Record, vol. i, 1889, p. 464..

taking exercises to improve her condition. Ferris waists, the equipoise waists or ribbon corsets offer the best substitutes for corsets.

TREATMENT OF DEVELOPED LATERAL CURVATURE.

Lateral curvature, being a condition usually that mani-

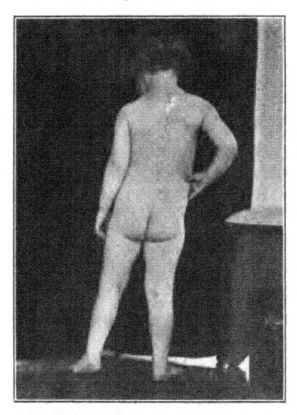

FIG. 98. THE SAME FAULTY ATTITUDE IN STANDING.

fests itself and is most active during the growing years of life, requires long and careful watching, which necessarily becomes trying to the parent and monotonous to the patient and surgeon, therefore treatment is difficult to enforce and results must necessarily vary with the degree of accord that exists between the patient and surgeon. As a consequence of this, no definite promises can be made as to the outcome of treatment, especially in bad cases and as it does not imperil life when untreated, as is the case in Pott's Disease, the patient has to go into it very earnestly, seriously, and persistently to hope for a good result and confidence in and obedience to the detailed treatment is essential. As a consequence of the tediousness and uncertainty of results, many physicians turn their cases over to Swedes or gymnasium instructors unskilled in "corrective work," without routine direction of the treatment and then to a large extent their responsibility ceases. The treatment, however, by these means may yield in mild cases good results, but are attained as a rule unscientifically, as the treatment is directed against the prominent shoulder, hips, or ribs and the primary causative condition, i. e., the deviated spine, is lost sight of. The treatment by orthopædic surgeons varies of course with the activity of the disease and its extent. It has three chief aims.

1. The removal of the superimposed weight resting on an habitual lateral deviation of the spine.

2. Strengthening and restoring the equilibrium in the osseous, ligamentous and muscular elements in the trunk.

3. To reduce or remove the deformity.

1. To remove the superimposed weight, two means are adopted, (a) recumbency and (b) suspension.

(a) Recumbency is one of the oldest forms of treatment and is most helpful in all cases and especially those in which the deformity is rapidly developing and where there is general weakness and slight endurance. The great objection, however, to it when prolonged is that when persisted in for months as an indoor treatment, the general health suffers and the conditions which promote the formation of solid bone and firm strong muscles are interfered with. Where

there are neurasthenic pains, however, recumbency carried
to the extent of several hours a day will be found most useful if supplemented with massage.   As a rule in all cases
where there is a tendency to be easily fatigued or a condition
of lowered vitality from too rapid growth, etc., recumbency
should be advised in the form of early retiring, late rising
and a period of afternoon recumbency more or less prolonged, depending on the severity of the case.

(b) Suspension as a rule means by the head and hands
equally without muscular effort.   To hang by the head only
has seemed severe and perhaps dangerous to the writer, but
in McKenzie's cases has proved efficient.[53]   The best means
for attaining suspension are by the ordinary head sling
attached to a rope passing over a pulley, the other end of
which has a cross bar of wood or knobs for the hands whereby
an equal distribution of weight can be maintained.   It goes
without saying that actual suspension for a prolonged period
is out of the question, but as a daily exercise either vertically or on an inclined plane, it does good in removing superincumbent weight and in lengthening muscles and ligaments
that have undergone adaptive shortening.   It may also
relieve the discomfort which is caused by the unequal distribution of the weight of the trunk on a weakened spine
with muscular contractions.   Exercises in swinging on the
trapeze may also do good in the same way.   By means of a
head support or "jury mast" partial suspension is obtainable
and is most beneficial in mild cervical and upper dorsal
cases and essential in some severe cases.   (Fig. 114.)   However, it is to be remembered, except in mild cases (and the
same holds in recumbency), that distraction by a direct pull
is no more efficient in obliterating a bad curve in true scoliosis

Trans., Amer. Orthop. Assoc., vol. vii.   Galloway: Annual Jour. Winnipeg
Medico Chirurgical Society, 1905–1906.

than in spondylitis, but simply removes the physiological curves, i. e., straightens them out.

2. The strengthening and restoration of the equilibrium in the trunk may be divided into its constituents for convenience, as (a) bone, (b) ligaments, (c) muscles.

(a) Bone development and strength must be gained by observing the laws of general hygiene by stimulating cold baths, exercises and fresh air and such diet and tonics as promote digestion, assimilation, etc.

Trabecular balance or equalization of strain on the two sides of the vertebræ must be gained according to Wolff's law by *over-correction* of the deformity in flexibles cases, as far as possible. (*vide infra.*)

(b) The ligaments are helped by such means as reëstablish the equilibrium, take the strain off one side and make the relaxed side bear its portion of the burden. These means are promoted by recumbency and suspension, by a drill in the proper attitude or by supports which hold the trunk erect or tend to over-correct the deformity. (*vide infra.*)

(c) *Muscles.* Under muscular improvement comes that most important subject of gymnastics, which should be employed in all cases of lateral curvature. Various authorities differ in the choice of exercises for the treatment of lateral curvature as one exercise in one man's hands may prove most efficient in a certain class of cases, while to another it may be of no value, as so much depends upon the way it is executed. All seem to concur in choosing exercises for increasing the flexibility and strength of the spinal column and muscular development of the shoulders and hips. In each case as it presents itself, the surgeon may find an exercise which has proven efficient in a similar case may not be useful in the one before him, and therefore the patient with back bared to the trochanters should be made to go through the various prescribed exercises in the surgeon's presence to determine their efficiency in each individual case. Thus the surgeon can write a prescription of exercises suited to the peculiar and particular requirements of the case. It is important also not to fatigue the patient by prolonged exercises and the movements at first should err on the side of being too short rather than the reverse, especially in those cases of lowered vitality and general debility. Thus will be apparent the unwisdom of class drills or exercises and the importance of treating the individual. Executing each motion from three to five times at the beginning will be found ample. Of great importance is the way in which a movement is executed, whether it brings into play the muscle or muscles desired, whether done *with a vim* or listlessly, or in a faulty attitude, or with knees or elbows bent when the reverse is essential, whether the correction aimed at is accomplished, etc. As a rule in mild cases a few exercises carefully executed twice daily will be found all that is necessary. In giving a list to a patient the exercises may be prescribed from a previously made lot of exercises which are adapted to cases in the different regions.

SWEDISH GYMNASTICS.

Gymnastic exercises in general are utilized for general muscular development but in lateral curvature, it is very essential to prescribe certain definite exercises to accomplish certain definite aims and each exercise should be done before the surgeon or his skilled gymnast to see that the scoliosis is helped thereby and in the case of a double curvature that one curve was not helped at the expense of another. Therefore it is most unwise, or at least a question of doubtful benefit, to send a scoliotic patient to a general gymnasium or to a gymnast unskilled in corrective work.

Hanging rings and pulley weights also are bad as allowing the hands to come close together and thus promote chest contraction.

However as many scoliotics are deficient in general muscular development, have insufficient or sluggish circulations and poor lung expansions, general gymnastic exercises carefully chosen must be prescribed to overcome these atonic conditions, as well as the special exercises to correct or lessen the curvatures.

Further, just as it is found in Pott's Disease that the more exaggerated the compensatory physiological curves became, the greater apparently is the deformity, so in scoliosis, we will find the greater the round shoulders or cervico-dorsal kyphosis and the greater the lumbar lordosis, the worse the scoliotic curves become. The converse of this is easily demonstrated by requesting a patient to hold the head up, chin in, chest out and abdomen back and at the same time overcome the lordosis by flexing the thighs on the body as in sitting or hanging in the "hook position" or in "hook lying" and then noting that the curvature is lessened somewhat. (Fig. 109.)

In order to carry out special or general Swedish movements for an individual case of scoliosis, but little apparatus is needed, viz: an inclined bar in a doorway, which can be made of a broomstick; a square stool of sufficient height to allow the patient's feet to rest squarely on the floor; a box of sufficient size to allow the patient to sit on it and gymnast to stand on it at the same time; a strip of wood with straps for the feet fastened obliquely against the chair-board and an oblong stool on a board sufficiently high for the patient to ride sitting astride thereon and have the feet fastened by straps to a board on the floor. For the specialist a regular Swedish boom, stall-bars, plinth, etc., will be most useful and one should refer to such special works as Anders Wide's Hand Book of Medical and Orthopædic Gymnastics[44] to get a thorough insight into this subject.

[44] Funk & Wagnalls Company, New York.

Swedish movements may be divided into active, passive and resisted movements: an active movement is one which the patient executes voluntarily by his or her own power; a passive movement is executed by the gymnast on some part of the patient's body and a movement with resistance may be either executed by the patient and resisted by the gymnast or executed by the gymnast and resisted by the patient, depending on the effect desired.

All Swedish movements are taken from what are termed fundamental positions, namely, in (1) standing, (2) sitting, (3) lying, or (4) hanging.

1. The standing fundamental position is with the head erect, chin in, chest out, abdomen in and hips drawn well back. The majority of Swedish books and gymnastic teachers require the patient to stand with the heels together and the long axes of the feet at 90° with each other. This is a weak position and detrimental to the arch of the foot, so that it is better to stand in what the Swedes call "close standing" with feet touching each other all along their inner sides or with their axes parallel at least. The arms hang freely at the sides with palms of hands against thighs and fingers close together.

2. In the sitting fundamental position the thighs are at a right angle to the trunk, the legs at 90° to thighs, the feet are firmly together on the floor and the knees together and the arms hang at the sides.

3. In lying the patient lies on the back, the arms are at the side, palms down and the legs are together, toes up.

4. In hanging the hands are *at least* as far apart as the width of the shoulders and the bar or trapeze is sufficiently high to prevent the toes from touching the ground. The arms are fully extended and the patient hangs passively.

From these fundamental positions innumerable movements or positions may be taken by combinations of definite arm, leg, or trunk attitudes.

ARM MOVEMENTS.

(*a*) In "wing" position, the hands are placed on the hips, fingers forward, thumb back.

(*b*) In "bend," the elbows are at the sides and finger tips touch the shoulders.

(*c*) In "swim," the elbows are on a level with the shoulders and radial side of hands toward shoulders.

(*d*) In "yard" or "cross c," the arms are fully extended laterally on a level with the shoulders.

(*e*) In "heave" or "cross e," arm rotation, the arms are on a level with the shoulders and the forearms at right angles with the arms, either forward or upward.

(*f*) In "reach," the entire arms are carried forward parallel to each other on a level with the shoulders; this is called "grasp" when the hands touch or rest on the wall or any apparatus. If the hands grasp anything this word is added for example, "reach-grasp-standing."

(*g*) "Rest" signifies that the palms of the hands rest on the back of the neck or head, so that the finger tips touch and the elbows are held well backward.

(*h*) "Stretch" means that the arms are fully extended upward.

"Half" signifies only one side is to execute a movement, but either "right" or "left" is more commonly used.

LEG MOVEMENTS.

(*a*) "Toe-standing" is where the patient stands on tip-toe.

(*b*) "Knee-bending," where the knees are flexed, and

(*c*) "Fall-out-standing" are the exercises chiefly used.

In "fall-out-standing," one foot is advanced forward about a yard, the knee is bent, so that it comes just over the toe-tips, the arm of that side is in the stretch position and with the body and the other fully extended leg, make one

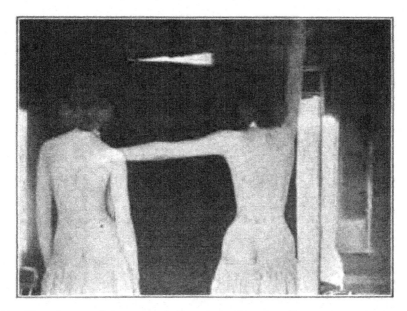

FIG. 99.   DOUBLE PHOTOGRAPHIC EXPOSURE. SHOWING DEFORMITY AND SELF-
CORRECTION IN A TOTAL LEFT DORSO-LUMBAR SCOLIOSIS BY THE "KEYNOTE."
POSITION IN THE SAME GIRL.

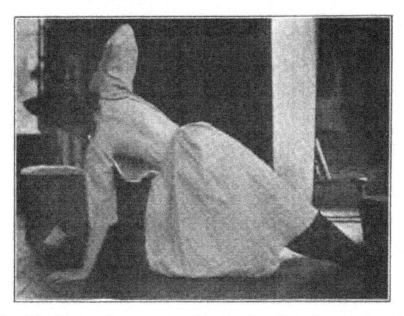

FIG. 100.   SIDEWAYS FALLING TO THE LEFT FOR LEFT DORSO-LUMBAR SCOLIOSIS.

plane; the other arm is carried downward and backward parallel to the upstretched arm.

"High-stepping" consists in tip-toeing, flexing the knees very high, walking forward, toes in or "marking time on the spot."

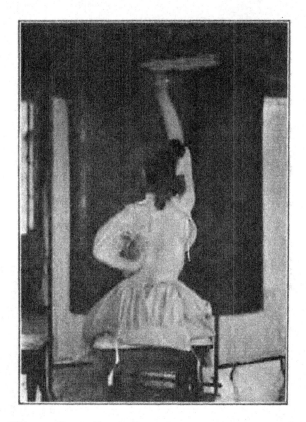

Fig. 101. "Sitting Right Reach Grasp Dumb-bell Left Press Over Ribs."

"Prone-standing" means flexing the body forward at the hip joints and not at the waist.

"Side bending" and "back bending" need no explanation.

"Leg-support-standing" means that the legs lean against or are supported by something.

"Forward" and "lateral-falling" mean positions in which the body is supported on the floor by the hands and feet, or one hand and one foot, respectively, with trunk and legs straight. (Fig. 100.)

SITTING POSITIONS.

The sitting positions, which have definite names as distinguished from the fundamental are: (Fig. 101.)

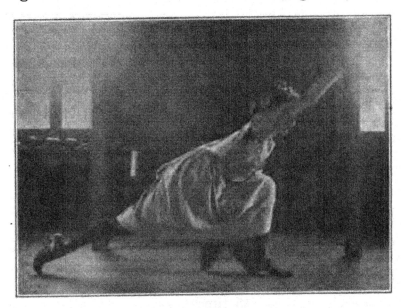

FIG. 102. "SPRING SITTING."

(a) "Long-sitting," where the legs are fully supported. (Fig. 83.)

(b) "Half-sitting" is where one thigh with knee flexed alone supports the weight of the body, the other leg being extended backward.

(c) "Stride sitting" is where the knees and feet are separated some little distance. (Fig. 81.)

(d) "Ride-sitting" is where the patient straddles or sits astride of some apparatus.

(e) "Spring-sitting" is practically the same thing as "fall-out-standing," with the flexed thigh supported on a stool, as a "half sitting" attitude modified. (Fig. 102.)

LYING POSITIONS.

(a) "Stride-lying" means the legs are separated.

(b) "Hook-lying" signifies the thighs are flexed on the body and the legs on the thighs. (Fig. 84.)

(c) "Sit-lying" means that the body and thighs are supported, but the legs depend as in sitting.

(d) "Half-lying" means the body lies at an angle of 45° on some supporting structure.

(e) "Hook-half-lying" combines (b) and (d).

(f) In "prone-lying" the patient lies on the face. (Fig. 78.)

(g) "Leg-prone-lying" means the legs rest on their anterior surface on some support. (Fig 79.)

(h) "Side-lying" and "side-leg-lying" need no explanation.

With these simple terms at our disposal, or combinations of them, covering exercises for the arms, legs and trunk, it is an easy matter to make out a programme for a case in brief language, for example, for general development, we might use.

1. Stretch-standing (15 times).

2. Yard-standing (15 times).

3. Heave-standing-arm rotation (15 times).

4. Rest, leg-prone-lying, holding (5 times).

5. Heave-hook-hanging.

6. Stretch, hook-half-lying, arm flexion and extension with resistance.

7. Toe-standing, knee-bending (25 times), etc.

FOR CERVICAL SCOLIOSIS.

1. Half yard-grasp-standing, head side flexion resisted toward the convexity.

2. Prone-lying, head bending backward resisted.

3. Lying, shoulder support, head twisting resisted (for rotation), etc.

FOR "c" SHAPED RIGHT DORSAL SCOLIOSIS.[55]

1. Left arm rest, right arm wing ride-sitting right side flexion.

2. Left spring-sitting.

3. Spinal-raising, which is a stretching position of the trunk from wing position.

4. Hanging, inclined boom (left side high). (Fig. 103.)

5. Left arm-stretch, right yard, toe standing, knee bending. (Left arm-stretch and right yard in right dorsal scoliosis is known as the "keynote" position or best position the patient can assume for straightening the curve.) (Fig. 99.)

6. Rest, prone-leg-lying, right side-bending, holding.

7. Left arm rest, right arm yard, side falling. (Fig. 100.)

8. Hook-hanging. (Fig. 109.)

9. Lying left leg raising (slowly) or prone-lying right leg extending slowly, resisted.

10. Hanging, fall out, left trunk twisting, etc.

FOR LUMBAR SCOLIOSIS (LEFT).

1. Standing right leg adduction or left hip lifting.

2. "Keynote" left side bending.

3. Prone-lying, double leg carrying to left.

4. Hanging double leg carrying to left.

5. Left side-falling, right arm rest, left arm grasp, stall-bars,[56] etc.

[55] In the illustrations it is to be noted the exercises are being given for *left* dorso-lumbar scoliosis. For the right curvature the exercises would be just reversed.

[56] Stall-bars or rib-stools as they are sometimes called, is a kind of ladder fastened against the wall.

For "S" formed scoliosis the exercises are to be so combined and adapted as to help both the dorsal and lumbar curves.

MECHANICAL CORRECTION.

The mechanical methods which are used to reduce or

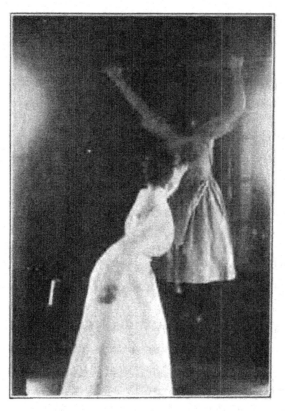

FIG. 103. HANGING, CORRECTION BY GYMNAST OF LEFT DORSO-LUMBAR SCOLIOSIS.

remove the deformity are: (1) To limit, prevent or check faulty attitudes, (2) to exert pressure over projecting ribs, shoulder or hip, and (3) to untwist the rotation and curves of the spine.

1. To limit, prevent or check faulty attitudes, elevation of one shoulder simply or even a flexible spinal curvature may be corrected by a strap passing around the shoulder on the side of the convexity, then down across the back to the opposite hip, where it is attached to a belt, which in turn is fastened to drawers or stockings or special thigh legging or perineal straps. A simple device of this kind was made of webbing and surgeon's plaster by the writer to over-correct

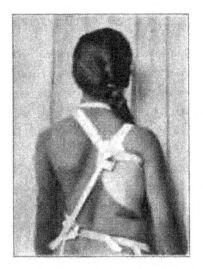

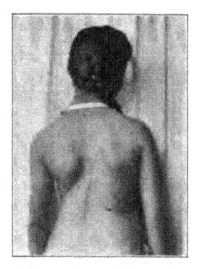

Fig. 104.   Fig 105.

FIG. 104. AUTHOR'S WEBBING CORRECTING BRACE.
FIG. 105. PATIENT BEFORE APPLICATION OF WEBBING BRACE.

the deformity in flexible cases as far as possible.[57] (Figs. 102 and 103.) He has found it the most useful form of light support and it is based on Wolff's law, and must be worn constantly except when doing routine gymnastics. If the other shoulder is lowered as well, a crutch may be attached to the belt to support it. Tilting of the pelvis or a lumbar curve should be helped by a tilted seat or a pad worn over

[57] Taylor: Amer. Jour. Orthop. Surg., Jan., 1905.

the buttock of the convex side in sitting or if one leg is short raising the sole of that shoe for walking and standing.

2. To exert pressure over projecting ribs, etc., various forms of braces have been used, utilizing the principles of tight straps, screw power and leverage, the last two, however, are not much used now, on account of their weight, which is an objection which will at once be apparent in a growing child already weak.

THE STEEL SCOLIOTIC BRACE.

The author devised and published the following scoliotic steel brace. A steel pelvic band is made with double perineal straps and has a steel upright extending up to the rotated ribs against which an adjustable plate attached to the upright presses. This upright by means of a ratchet arrangement and setscrews could be moved inward to exert more pressure on the laterally deviated trunk or vice versa. With bending irons the forward pressure against the projecting ribs could be increased by the spring force of the steel. On the front of the pelvic band at a point diagonally opposite the posterior upright, an anterior upright and pressure plate was similarly adjusted to afford counter-pressure against the projecting ribs. An axillary crutch attached to the pelvic band was sometimes found useful to support the low shoulder. This brace will be found useful in larger children in flexible and partially flexible curvatures in conjunction with gymnastic treatment.[58] (Fig. 106.)

THE CORRECTED PLASTER OF PARIS JACKET.

In the more severe partially flexible and fixed cases nothing will be found as useful as a removable plaster jacket made over a corrected plaster image of the body. This

[58] Taylor. N. Y. Med. Jour., vol. lxvi, Oct. 30, 1897.

method was first suggested by Bartow and modified by Bradford and Brackett.

The method now used at the Hospital for Crippled and Deformed Children consists briefly in measuring the circumferences of the thorax at axillæ and bust, waist and pel-

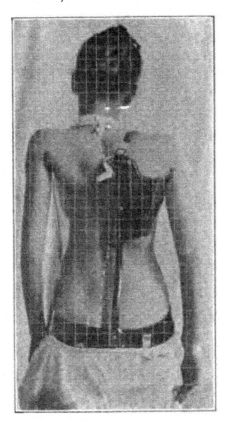

FIG. 106. THE AUTHOR'S STEEL SCOLIOSIS BRACE. PATIENT SAME AS IN FIG. 89.

vis of the patient; then the distances of the mammæ from the anterior superior spines. The patient then sits on a table to flex the thighs and overcome the lordosis as much as possible, a head sling is put on and the spine is stretched; the arms are supported to be on a level with the shoulders and

if much lateral leaning or twisting of the trunk exists efforts
are made to correct these by position as much as possible
or by pressure rods in the Hoffa machine. (*vide infra.*)
Over a suitable undershirt, without felt padding, a plaster
jacket is applied, which when dry is cut off and used as a
mold and filled with semi-liquid plaster of paris. This when
set gives us a duplicate of our patient.

A line is drawn joining the posterior superior spines and
upon the center of this is drawn a perpendicular line which
should be the line of the spinous processes. If the trunk is
found to lean markedly to one side, the inclination is determined with the vertical and a reverse or over-corrected
inclination is marked on the plaster for the future corrected
cast.

With a carpenter's draw knife the plaster cast is cut away
on the side of the convexity, both in regard to lateral lean
and rotation, front and back, and built up with semi-solid
plaster of paris on the concavity by wetting the set cast
previous to its application. Additional plaster is put over
the mammæ and anterior superior spines. The whole is
then smoothed, sandpapered and shellaced.

Comparison is then made with the original measurements
of the patient and if found to correspond, a plaster jacket is
made on this corrected cast over an undershirt with felt
pads over the anterior superior spines. When dry it is cut
down the front, removed and finished with an outside covering of stockinet and lacing, after thoroughly baking to remove
all moisture and render it as light as possible. (Fig. 107.)

Such a jacket, when worn by the patient, acts as a constantly correcting force to lessen lateral leaning and rotation.
It should be worn all the time except when going through
the gymnastics.

The author's experience with celluloid jackets made in
this manner is unsatisfactory in that they twist out of shape,

are very tedious and expensive to make and are hot even when well perforated with apertures.

The enameled paper jackets as advocated by Weigel and made over the corrected casts are too hot for the southern climate aside from their expense.

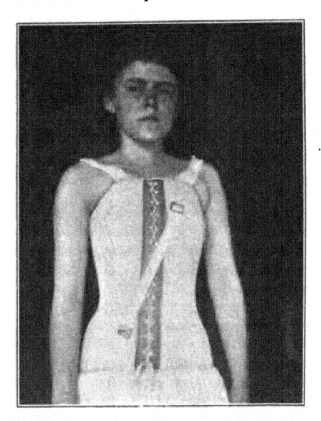

FIG. 107.   A PLASTER JACKET MADE OVER A CORRECTED CAST FOR A CASE OF SCOLIOSIS.

The same may be said of leather jackets and Phelp's aluminium corsets.

When a patient gets a very expensive jacket she is unwilling to discard it when further improvement prompts the surgeon to further correct the cast and make a new and more nearly normal jacket. So that in the long run a light, laced, cool and comparatively inexpensive plaster jacket is the best, in the author's judgment.

There are those who maintain that no brace, corset or support should be applied in scoliosis as weakening the muscles and others hold and can show the advantages clinically, that it is essential and mechanically sensible to hold a deviated spine as erect as possible by day and night for the more it leans to one side, the greater to a certain extent will be the tendency of gravity and pathological function to increase the deformity, but the muscles must be taken care of in these cases by having the patient do her exercises twice daily vigorously, without the jacket and have massage to the entire trunk if possible.

(3) The machines used to untwist the rotation and curves of the spine are:

(a) The Hoffa twister, which has the newest modifications as suggested by Weigel and Bradford and differs considerably from Hoffa's original. It consists of a steel arch, a head sling and adjustable hand supports, with pads for screw pressure to be exerted over the ribs and clamps for the hips. Hoffa's newest modification has a seat to overcome lordosis and raise either side of the pelvis desired. By means of this daily in a standing or sitting position from fifteen to thirty minutes in each case, pressure should be exerted to correct the lateral deviation of the spine and untwist the rotation of the ribs. (Fig. 108.)

(b) The modified Lorenz roller is a padded roller on which the prominent ribs of the patient's back rests as she stands on the floor, the arm of that side surrounds the roller and the hand of the concave side grasps a bar, which can be moved by a crank and raise the patient from the ground, causing the weight of the entire body to exert pressure on the prominent ribs against the padded roller. By lying with the prominent side on the roller, the spinal curve can be temporarily straightened and the shortened ligaments stretched daily.

(c) The Zander rocker is a machine on which the patient lies. It is divided in the middle by a pad against which the

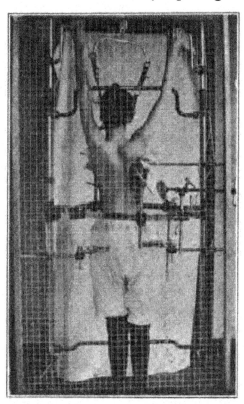

FIG. 108. HOFFA'S TWISTER.

prominent ribs rest. The arms are extended upward and grasp a strap. The lower part is balanced by a weight and hinged so that the patient can be rocked up and down and increase the flexibility of the spine by daily stretching.

(d) Riely's modification of Beely's pressure machine consists of two padded supports for the upper thorax and pelvis on which the patient rests face down with the thigh flexed at right angles with the trunk to lessen the lordosis. A strap passes over the rotated ribs at the point of greatest curvature, one end of the strap is made fast to the wall and on the other hooks are provided to put weights on up to 100 pounds, which is often not found too much pressure for these cases. By raising the wall attachment of the strap greater correction is effected in the lateral curvature and by lowering it the rotation is chiefly reduced.

In Beely's machine, the patient's trunk is unsupported save by the arms and legs and fatigue is much sooner experienced.

These machines may be employed in the daily routine of treatment, with benefit.

FORCIBLE CORRECTION.

Certain cases of moderately severe grade are best treated by solid plaster of paris jackets put on in some machine which can effect more or less forcible correction. This can be done in the Hoffa machine or either of the two following. By this means if these jackets are changed every two or three weeks, a progressive stretching of the contracted ligaments and muscles may be effected and if persisted in for a sufficiently long period the bones too will undergo functional transformation. Later gymnastics, massage and the wearing of removable plaster jackets made over a corrected cast will accomplish much.

(e) The writer's machine[50] is a modification of the large supine recumbent kyphotone, with the addition of hemispherical arcs to which are attached screw pressure rods and plates similar to those used in the Hoffa machine. (Figs. 110, 111 and 112.)

The pelvis is supported by a crutch and the thorax by the lateral and diagonal antero-posterior pressure rods. Trac-

[50] Johns Hopkins Hospital Bulletin, No. 45, February, 1895.

tion on the head is made by the ordinary head sling and double pulleys, the hands grasp the hand rods and the legs are made fast to the stirrups. Then as much forcible correction as possible is made by the pressure rods and traction, and a corrective plaster jacket is applied.

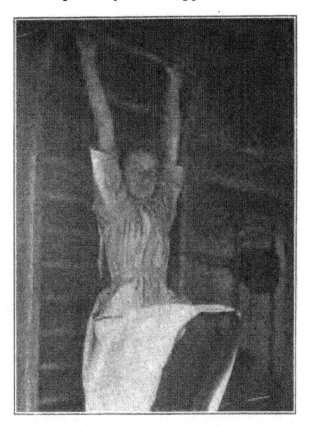

FIG. 109. HOOK HANGING.

(f) In certain instances as demonstrated by Lovett in his experiments[60] more correction by side pressure can be obtained by *not* using traction on the spine, just as one could bend a stick more readily if traction, which resists the lateral forces, is not made on the two ends.

[60] Boston Medical and Surgical Journal, March 17, 1904.

Lovett's experiments were made with flexible rods, cadaver and healthy living subjects and in each the side pull was more marked without traction than with it.

On these facts the Lovett-Adams machine was constructed. It consists of a pelvic support and clamps; the body is prone and the thighs are at a right angle to the body, which is surrounded by three double circles with two pressure rods each, on each central circle, which may be made to rotate or not by a setscrew on the outer circle. (Fig. 113.)

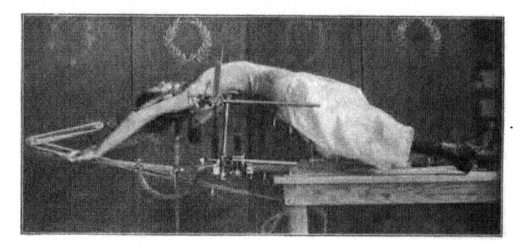

FIG. 110. AUTHOR'S SCOLIOSIS CORRECTION MACHINE.

The pelvic support and circles rest on a gaspipe frame.

Pressure is made directly and not obliquely on the lateral inclination of the trunk and rotation of the ribs or the lateral inclination is corrected by lateral movement of the entire circular segment on the gaspipe frame; then the deformed spine is derotated in the desired direction at the three different segments by moving the circles. When the desired degree of correction is obtained a fixed plaster of paris jacket is applied. Such a jacket is worn two weeks then removed, and more correction tried and so on. Later the same after-treatment is employed as with the Hoffa machine. In upper dorsal and cervical scoliosis traction must be used and the head and neck included in plaster or some steel brace or jacket and jury mast employed. (Fig. 114.)

(g) *Table and Strap Pulley Machine.* This simple piece of apparatus was devised at the Children's Hospital, Boston, and is based upon Lovett's experiments also.

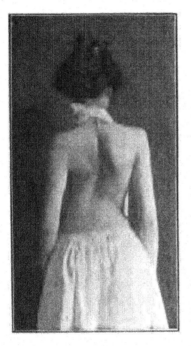 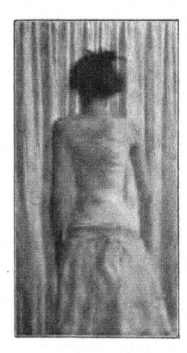

FIG. 111. FIG. 112.

FIG. 111. PATIENT SHOWN IN 110, BEFORE APPLICATION OF FORCIBLE CORRECTION.
FIG. 112. PATIENT SHOWN IN 111 AFTER CORRECTION.

It consists of an ordinary kitchen table into the center of one end of which is screwed a hook to which is attached a compound pulley. On the sides of the opposite end are four or five cleats at intervals.

The patient kneels on a stool at this end and the trunk lies prone between the two rows of cleats. By means of an encircling webbing strap and attached cords the pelvis is made fast to a cleat on the side of the maximum convexity. In the same manner a strap makes fast the highest part of the thorax under the axillæ when the arms are fully extended upward. On the side of the concavity a pulley is fastened to a cleat and a cord passes to the lower side of a strap which

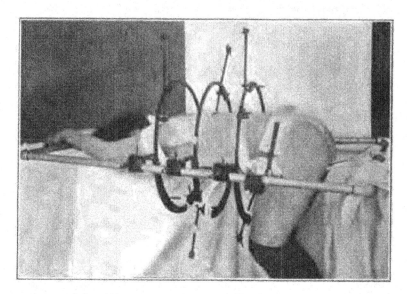

FIG. 113. LOVETT ADAMS' FORCIBLE CORRECTION MACHINE.

should encircle the trunk at this point, the upper side of which is made fast to a cleat near the pulley. The cord which passes through the pulley goes to the lower one of the compound pulleys. By a cord from the upper compound pulley the patient or gymnast can not only effect lateral correction of the curvature, but derotation of the trunk as well in flexible and partially flexible cases.

We also use a segmented table devised by Lovett with a central axis and straps arranged very much as in the above apparatus and it possesses only the advantage that the segments may be rotated with the aim of untwisting the spine and has rachetted pressure pads for lateral and posterior curves.

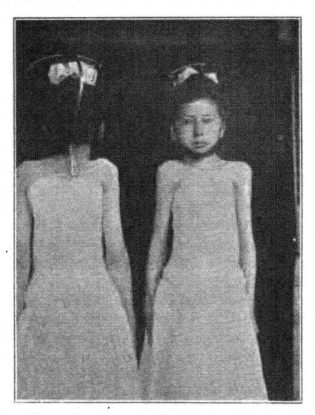

Fig. 114. A Jury Mast Worn with Plaster Jacket in Severe Cervico-Dorsal Scoliosis.

These last two machines, however, are used only for daily routine correction and not as a means of obtaining correction while a plaster jacket is being applied.

SUMMARY

The summary of treatment that may be employed is:

1. In incipient postural cases, where curves disappear with

recumbency and suspension, postural treatment with preventive measures should be used.

2. When in addition to the above, muscular weakness and habitually faulty attitudes are present corrective gymnastics must be used in addition.

3. In "flexible" curves that are becoming rapidly more pronounced fixative appliances to over-correct the deformity have practical as well as scientific value.

4. In partly "fixed" curves, where more or less muscular, ligamentous and osseous changes have taken place, daily methodical correction for several months or even years together with corrective gymnastics, suspension, recumbency and fixative strapping or jackets must be resorted to.

5. In "fixed" cases that are not hopelessly deformed forcible correction is very helpful and may be obtained by means of the author's machine, the Hoffa twister, or the Lovett-Adams apparatus when a fixed series of jackets are to be applied. Subsequently the case is to be treated as a partly fixed curvature.

Daily corrective gymnastics are extremely valuable in all cases until ossification is complete and prolonged recumbency at mid-day with early retiring, late rising and a cold morning sponge bath should be insisted on for these relaxed girls.

The time required for treatment is in the growing years, in light cases with weekly, monthly, quarterly or semi-annual inspections and instructions and in the severer and apparently increasing cases with methodical daily corrections by gymnastics, machines and fixative appliances.

INDEX.

INDEX.

CPSIA information can be obtained at www.ICGtesting.com
Printed in the USA
BVOW09s1015270415

397857BV00015B/240/P